ACCESSIBLE YOGA

POSES AND PRACTICES FOR EVERY BODY

Jivana Heyman

Foreword by Matthew Sanford
Photos by Sarit Z. Rogers

SHAMBHALA
BOULDER
2019

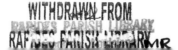

Shambhala Publications, Inc.
4720 Walnut Street
Boulder, Colorado 80301
www.shambhala.com

The content of this book is not intended as medical advice. Please seek approval from your health care practitioner before attempting any of the methods described here.

The names and details of students described have been changed to protect their privacy.

9 8 7 6 5 4 3 2 1

First Edition
Printed in the United States of America

⊛This edition is printed on acid-free paper that meets the American National Standards Institute Z39.48 Standard.
♻Shambhala Publications makes every effort to print on recycled paper. For more information please visit www.shambhala.com.
Shambhala Publications is distributed worldwide by Penguin Random House, Inc., and its subsidiaries.

Designed by Gopa&Ted2, Inc.

Library of Congress Cataloging-in-Publication Data
Names: Heyman, Jivana, author.
Title: Accessible yoga: poses and practices for every body / Jivana Heyman;
    foreword by Matthew Sanford; photos by Sarit Rogers.
Description: First edition. | Boulder: Shambhala, 2019. | Includes
    bibliographical references and index.
Identifiers: LCCN 2019004002 | ISBN 9781611807127 (paperback: alk. paper)
Subjects: LCSH: Yoga. | Yoga—Therapeutic use.
Classification: LCC RA781.67 .H49 2019 | DDC 613.7/046—dc23
LC record available at https://lccn.loc.gov/2019004002

For my mother

CONTENTS

FOREWORD

WHEN I STARTED practicing yoga in 1991, I got extraordinarily lucky. There was no path to follow, no signposts, no whispers in ancient texts, and no how-to book. There was no Internet flush with magical search engines, no social media posts, no Instagram, and no Facebook. I was lucky enough to meet an amazing, big-hearted Iyengar yoga teacher named Jo Zukovich. We didn't know what to do, but she was confident enough to make me a partner in a great experiment. We explored yoga and disability together.

In 1978, at age thirteen, I was injured in a car accident that killed my father and sister and rendered me completely paralyzed from the chest down. By the time I started practicing yoga twelve years later, I was sick of the Western medical model. I was sick of doctors, of interventions, of physical and occupational therapy, of always being treated like a patient by everyone just because I was disabled. Thankfully, Jo didn't do this. She did not let fear of my "otherness" get in the way of our yogic study. She helped me become a yoga student just like any other yoga student, except different.

The fact is that yoga, and in particular asana, looks different when it travels through my paralyzed body. On the outside, my poses rarely look as they would if I were a "traditional" yoga student (whatever that is). On the inside, however, my poses are forged with the timeless heart of yoga. The principles of yoga and asana do not discriminate. Yoga poses do, that is, unless the poses are made accessible to all comers. This simple insight led me to become a yoga teacher, found the nonprofit Mind Body Solutions, and dedicate my life to opening yoga for everyone

This is a vision that I share with Jivana Heyman, the author of this book. Jivana came to the importance of making yoga accessible to all from a different path than I did. Beginning as a social activist, he has been advocating for equal and fair treatment for all people throughout his adult life. At heart, I believe Jivana experienced the healing power of yoga in his own life and is now working to ensure that potential for everyone. He is a man of service with one of the kindest hearts and noblest visions that I have encountered.

I have watched him work tirelessly, building not just his organization and trainings, but an international movement aiming to open the door of yoga in all directions and to all people. What's not to like?

The sacred heart of yoga is inclusive, giving, and ultimately offers transcendent healing to everyone willing to practice. With this book, Jivana has done an enormous service. He has created a runway to the healing potential of yoga for all people. This is the book I needed back in 1991. It would have given me the courage to begin. It also would have helped me know that I was not alone, that someone does in fact care about the potential yoga students not living in the mainstream. Most important, this book would have helped me know that I belong in the ever-growing community of yogis both past and present.

—Matthew Sanford

ACKNOWLEDGMENTS

I'M TAKING the unusual step of starting to write this book with the acknowledgments, because it could not have happened without the love and dedication of so many people. The Accessible Yoga movement has grown into something I could never have imagined, and there are so many people to thank for that. So many people that I can't begin to thank them all—although this will be a very long and very incomplete list!

I have to begin with my husband, Matt, who after twenty-five years, is still loving and patient with me. And our children, Charlie and Violet, who are my teachers.

This book is dedicated to my mother, who died recently, and to her passion for books, which always inspired me to want to write one. I'm so glad that she knew about this project before she passed. It's also dedicated to my father; my stepmother, Judy; my siblings, Jenny and Mike, Tim, Chris and Anna, and Amanda and Greg; and my uncle Gary, cousin Alexa, and nieces and nephews; and my in-laws, Rick and Charlie.

Special thanks to Sarit Rogers for her amazing photographs. She has the innate ability to capture both the spiritual and political with her camera. And she can do so in a captivating way that makes you feel comfortable and grounded as a subject and as a viewer. Thank you to De Jur Jones, the main model for the book. She is a powerful teacher who is able to transmit the essence of yoga through her very being. Thank you Melanie Williams for your amazing support during this process.

The idea for this book was crafted with Kathleen Kraft and Mary Beth Ray. Special thanks to my writing support team: Linda Sparrowe, for her passion, and Nina Zolotow, for her clarity. Some of these writings also appeared in Yoga International's website, and I'm very grateful for the organization's support. In particular, I want to thank Kat Heagberg for her editing and handstand skills.

I am so grateful to Beth Frankl, Breanna Locke, Peter Schumacher, Karen Steib, and the entire Shambhala Publications team. You made this easy, and that's saying a lot!

Accessible Yoga is in many ways a child of Integral Yoga and the AIDS epidemic. Integral Yoga is the school my teacher Swami Satchidananda created when he came to the United States in the sixties. When he arrived, he saw that Westerners needed an adapted yoga practice, and that's what he created. I'm so grateful to him and to all my teachers who helped me understand the nature of yoga: Kazuko Onodera, Swami Vimalananda, Swami Karunananda, Swami Asokananda, Swami Divyananda, Swami Vidyananda, Swami Suddhananda, Swami Sarvaananda, Nischala Joy Devi, Jnani Chapman, Vidya Vonne, Arturo Peal, Sonia Sumar, Eric Small, and many others.

Thank you to my mentors and dear friends Swami Ramananda and Cheri Clampett, who support me endlessly and listen to me patiently. Their guidance has been invaluable.

This book is also dedicated to all those teachers who were out there making yoga accessible long before I came along. People like Matthew Sanford, who pioneered this work. What an honor to have him write the foreword! Teachers like Kalyani Baral, Ana Killingstat, Prakasha Capen, Judith Hanson Lasater, Donna Farhi, Lakshmi Voelker, JoAnn Lyons, Richard Rosen, Durga Leela, Molly Lannon Kenny, Haris Lender, Sarahjoy Marsh, Hamsa Spagnola, Stacie Dooreck, Willem Wittstamm, Satya Greenstone, Baxter Bell, Mukunda and Chinnamasta Stiles, and so many others.

I feel so grateful to the expert contributors to this book who are the force behind the growth of this work in the world. There is detailed information about them at the end of the book.

Accessible Yoga wouldn't exist without the love and dedication of our board: Priya Wagner (who started it all), Sarani Fedman, Prashanti Goodell, Amber Karnes, Mary Sims, Kerri Hanlon, Matthew Taylor, and previous board members Dianne Bondy, Rudra Swartz, and Steffany Moonaz. Our staff—Megan Zander, Brina Lord, Sevika Ford, Kelly Palmer, and Sarah Helt—make the magic happen.

Special thanks to Maitreyi Picerno and Ian Waisler, who shared this vision with me from the very beginning. Plus, all our Accessible Yoga Ambassadors around the world who are working every day to make yoga available to people who don't have access to these life-changing practices. This book is dedicated to you.

Thank you to the following for your support and inspiration: Prem Anjali, Felicia Tomasko, Danica Hodge, Melanie Klein, Chandra Sgammato, Robert

McLoud, Lakshmi Sutter, Hersha Harilela, David Lipsius, Matthew Remski, Seth Powell, Kamala Demaris, Uma Cocchi, Anna Fandino, Shakti Bell, Tim O'Toole, Mike Iveson, Nancy Solomon, Kristie Dahlia Home, Brenda Bakke, and Mary Fuhr. Thank you to Barbara Hirsch, Sarah Tuttle, Holly Rushing, and my Santa Barbara Yoga Center family, who are grateful for me even though I never come to work!

I also want to thank all my students, who have been so generous to share their practice with me. This book is the result of what I learned from you.

INTRODUCTION
My Story

MY ACCESSIBLE YOGA story began in the early 1990s. I was living in San Francisco right after college. I had come out of the closet at seventeen, and that's when my life suddenly opened up. I found a new excitement and hopefulness that I'd lost in my closeted adolescent days. I was experiencing a freedom I'd never known. Although that freedom came from being out, it was actually an internal experience that came from accepting myself for who I am.

The voices of self-hatred and self-criticism that had haunted me were quieted by a blossoming self-love. So moving to San Francisco, the gay mecca, seemed like the beginning of a new chapter for me. Unfortunately, rather than finding the carefree life I had imagined, I found myself surrounded by a world of illness and death because so many of my friends were getting sick and dying of AIDS.

AIDS offered a quick lesson in the most painful aspects of our human condition. While most twenty-year-olds were out having fun, I found myself marching in the streets with ACT UP (The AIDS Coalition to Unleash Power), volunteering at an AIDS hospice, and working for an underground AIDS newsletter.

One of the patients at the AIDS hospice where I volunteered, John, was about the same age as me, in his early twenties, and near death. He was so angry about dying that he wouldn't allow any of the hospice volunteers to come into his room other than to bring the food he could barely eat. He would just yell at them to leave him alone. When I started to volunteer, the staff thought John might be willing to talk to another young person. So they sent me to try to talk to him. I was afraid to enter his room because he yelled at all the other volunteers and was angry all the time. Eventually, I got up the courage, and John hesitatingly let me come in. He even teased me about it and asked if I thought I was a saint for coming to visit him. He had a sharp wit and equally sharp tongue that seemed unimpaired even as his body failed.

We got into a routine, and I would visit him a few days a week. Most of the time John would rant about how angry he was about being sick and talk about how much he wanted to be out having fun. He grilled me for details about my life out in the world. Where did I go, who did I see? I remember feeling guilty for having a social life. I did my best to listen to his anger and fear and try not to get too caught up in it myself. But it was impossible.

I remember one time John was so angry he stood up on his bed, almost naked, jumping up and down screaming like a child having a temper tantrum. The reason he wasn't wearing any clothes was because his body was covered with open sores that wouldn't heal, and his clothing was sticking to the sores making them more painful. It was impossible to witness his suffering without getting angry myself. I was furious with a world that didn't care about John and his pain. And it was an anger I held on to for many years.

This anger carried me through years of protesting in the streets with ACT UP and getting arrested for civil disobedience on many occasions. One time a small group of us chained ourselves to the inside of a subway train during rush hour in San Francisco in an attempt to gain attention for our loved ones who were getting sick and dying. Looking back, it seems so extreme, but I was completely committed to serving those who were suffering. My anger was the only outlet I had.

Anger can be useful when facing oppression, but anger unchecked can do a lot of damage. I was having serious stress-related digestive problems and stumbled into a yoga class with a teacher named Kazuko Onodera. I found myself returning week after week. I was reminded of some of my earliest childhood memories, which were watching my grandmother practice yoga every morning. Slowly the yoga crept up on me. What seemed like simple stretching, breathing, and relaxing was actually transforming me. Without realizing it, I was growing and healing.

After some time, I went to an ACT UP protest where there was a counter demonstration going on. The two groups were on either side of a single metal police barricade yelling at each other. I noticed two men at the front, standing on either side of the barricade, who were screaming at each other furiously. Both men were red-faced and fuming. In that moment, I realized that in their anger these two men were basically the same. It dawned on me that in my anger I could only accomplish so much. I was tired of yelling and screaming, when what I really wanted was to help my friends heal.

I slowly started backing away from the crowd and walked away down the street. The noise from the yelling lingered in my ears. As I walked away from the demonstration that day, I began to feel the deep sadness and loss that were at the root of my anger. The anger had been covering up my grief over the loss of my friends and the loss of my innocence.

When the anger dissipated, I realized that there was something else I could do. I could share yoga with my community. I could support my friends with the powerful practices of yoga as they struggled with illness and death.

From the outside, yoga may seem self-indulgent and exclusive. But much of what we think of yoga is really a modern, Westernized practice. At its heart, yoga is about love and service, not yoga pants and Instagram followers. Yoga wasn't stopping me from being an AIDS activist—it was showing me how to be a more effective one. In fact, yoga is designed to amplify our voices by giving us tools to make us stronger and clearer. It's designed to make us peaceful warriors. We can use yoga to deepen our connection to love and truth; to speak up for those who don't have a voice.

WHAT IS HEALING?

I graduated from yoga teacher training just weeks before my best friend, Kurt, died of AIDS in 1995. Kurt's death cemented my commitment to sharing yoga with the AIDS community. After graduation, I immediately started a yoga class for people with HIV/AIDS at the Integral Yoga Institute in San Francisco.

I also started teaching a similar class at a local hospital, and the classes began to grow. Students with other disabilities began asking if they could join. I soon found myself teaching yoga to people with all different disabilities around the San Francisco Bay Area.

Eventually, I got a job teaching yoga for the Dean Ornish Heart Disease Reversal Program. Dr. Ornish's research showed that the yoga lifestyle could reverse heart disease, the leading cause of death for both men and women around the world. Everyone seemed to focus on the extremely low-fat vegetarian diet he recommended, but what was most incredible was that he had scientifically proven that yoga heals. He also discovered that two components of his program were particularly effective: the more time the patients spent practicing yoga and participating in support groups, the healthier they got.[1]

Those two things, yoga and community, became the theme of my work going forward. I worked to bring that same support group feeling into my HIV/AIDS yoga classes by adding a short time in each class for sharing and discussion. Sometimes we would read yoga philosophy or poetry; sometimes we would just talk about how we were feeling.

This created a very strong bond and kept the same group of students coming back year after year. I remember one student named Gordon, who had been coming to the class at the hospital for a few years. He would share his struggles with his health and alcohol, and he would joke about how he wasn't a good yogi. He also loved when we shared poetry, especially a Rumi poem called "Love Dogs."

One day Gordon told the group that he had been diagnosed with pancreatic cancer, which may have been related to his AIDS diagnosis. He told us he only had a few months to live. A few weeks later, one of the other students found out that Gordon had been admitted to the same hospital where we had our class. So that day, we all decided to go visit him in his room upstairs instead of doing yoga.

We sat around Gordon's hospital bed making small talk. Then he asked if I would read his favorite poem. Luckily I had the poetry book with me, and as I read the poem, I could see his eyes glowing. I was amazed that he could be so physically ill but seem so peaceful and so connected. Gordon died a few days later, and our class mourned his loss. But we were so happy that we were able to spend that moment together with Gordon, and we were all grateful to him for showing us how true healing is possible even in death.

LOVE DOGS

One night a man was crying,
Allah! Allah!
His lips grew sweet with the praising,
until a cynic said,
"So! I have heard you
calling out, but have you ever
gotten any response?"

The man had no answer to that.
He quit praying and fell into a confused sleep.

He dreamed he saw Khidr, the guide of souls,
in a thick, green foliage.
"Why did you stop praising?"
"Because I've never heard anything back."
"This longing
you express *is* the return message."

The grief you cry out from
draws you toward union.

Your pure sadness
that wants help
is the secret cup.

Listen to the moan of a dog for its master.
That whining is the connection.

There are love-dogs
no one knows the names of.

Give your life
to be one of them.[2]
—RUMI

I thought a lot about the message of that poem, the idea that "the grief you cry out from draws you toward union." It's our challenges that bring us to yoga. Our pain that forces us to grow. I slowly started to understand that teaching yoga isn't about healing other people. Instead, it's about giving people access to the yoga practices and creating community to support that practice. Teaching yoga is about creating a safe space for people to explore themselves. And it's one of life's great ironies that the source of our healing is our own pain and suffering—even our anger.

What does healing really mean if we are all going to get sick and eventually die? Healing is often proclaimed as a transformation to some idealized physical state, but that's really an illusion, isn't it? In fact, the illusion of perfect health is one of the things that actually interferes with healing.

Isn't healing really a process of reconnecting or making whole? The word *healing* means to make whole and is similar to the Sanskrit word *yoga*, which also means to unite or make whole. Really, yoga—and healing—are about forging a strong inner connection. This healing may or may not coincide with physical healing. In fact, it's possible to be healed and to die.

WHO DESERVES YOGA?

Economic status, race, sexuality, gender identity, and ability can all limit access to opportunity. Although life can be challenging for everyone, our personal privilege will often predict how much money and physical comfort life brings. It will also limit access to quality health care and self-care practices like yoga. To practice yoga, you need access to yoga teachers and information about yoga. You need the time and money to go to class, buy a book, or get a subscription to an online service. You also need to believe that yoga is an appropriate practice for you.

Unfortunately, most yoga spaces are not welcoming to people with disabilities, fat students, or anyone who doesn't fit the commercial image of the yoga practitioner. How do we change this limited understanding of who can practice yoga? We can start by exploring what yoga really is.

Yoga is an interesting term. In Sanskrit, the word *yoga* has more meanings than any other word. It's a diverse group of practices from many different ancient and not-so-ancient traditions in India. At its heart, yoga is a spiritual practice that can be used by anyone at any time—if you know how. Yoga is a path of self-exploration, self-study, and self-awareness.

Yoga is not a replacement for basic human rights, as I'll discuss later. But yoga teaches another way to look at life. Rather than putting all our energy into externally focused pursuits, yoga shows us that there is tremendous benefit in cultivating our internal lives. Ultimately, what we are looking for is found inside. When we relax the body and breath, and start making friends with the mind, we may experience a shift. This is the goal of yoga: shifting our focus from outward to inward.

Making this internal shift is challenging for everyone, regardless of ability. It doesn't matter if you can stand on your head or not. In fact, there is no correlation between physical ability and peace of mind. People who seem to have it all can be miserable. People with disabilities or chronic illness, those who have suffered trauma or discrimination, and people who have been marginalized all have equal claim to the peace of yoga.

In fact, the most powerful tools of yoga, like breathing practices and meditation, are actually the most subtle and most accessible. For example, meditation works directly with the mind, teaching us how to let go of stress and detach from our obsessive thinking. *Yoga nidra* is a powerful form of guided meditation that leads us on an inner journey to the deeper layers of our being. *Pranayama*, the breathing practices, gives us ways to direct energy and soothe the mind. These subtle, accessible practices do not rely on gymnastic ability or great physical strength. In fact, most do not rely on gross physical movement at all! What a relief that anyone can access these tools, the most powerful yoga practices.

I remember one yoga student named Tanya, who used to come to a class I led for people with multiple sclerosis (MS) through an outpatient clinic in San Francisco. She taught me a huge lesson about yoga, meditation, and how to find peace. Tanya had quadriplegia from advanced multiple sclerosis, meaning her body was mostly immobile. She had very limited movement in her face and hands. Also, her speech was slow, and she had to take a breath between each phrase. Otherwise, she was completely paralyzed.

Tanya lived in a county-run hospital serving people who had advanced disabilities and no money or support system. Our yoga class was at a different hospital on the other side of town. She arranged for the disability transport service to pick her up and bring her to class every week. The transport agency would give her a three-hour window for when they would pick her up and for when they would take her home. For the one-hour yoga class, she would spend up to three hours waiting for them to bring her to class. Then, after class, she would wait up to three hours more for them to pick her up. It was a full-day affair!

Remarkably, Tanya seemed undisturbed by this situation and would happily return to class week after week. As I got to know her better, I found she was a very relaxed and content person, despite her physical condition. It was a revelation to me. The idea of being completely immobile scared me, and I couldn't imagine being in Tanya's situation myself, without constantly fighting off depression. Yet she seemed content.

After a few months of coming to class, she asked me a question about meditation. I had been teaching the class to use a mantra, Japa Yoga, instructing them to repeat the mantra OM SHANTI. I explained that "OM" represents the sound of the entire universe, and "SHANTI" means peace. Tanya admitted, "I have been trying to repeat OM SHANTI, but I can't seem to focus on it for very long."

I immediately started lecturing her about how meditation can be challenging and how it is normal for the mind to wander—my normal canned meditation talk. But she continued, "Instead, my mind keeps going back to the Lord's Prayer, which I'm constantly repeating." I stood there amazed and then laughed at my assumptions.

In effect, Tanya was experiencing a deep meditation with her mind focused on the Lord's Prayer all the time. I told her how beautiful that was and how she shouldn't worry about repeating OM SHANTI but continue with her practice. She was meditating successfully, and it was obviously bringing her great peace and comfort. Even in such a difficult physical situation, the repetition of a prayer or mantra can be transformative. Tanya showed me how effective the subtle practice of meditation is and how someone with almost no physical ability could still be a great yogi. Tanya's practice is a great example of the power of meditation which we will discuss and explore in chapter 13.

TOWARD AN ACCESSIBLE YOGA

In a way, the story of Accessible Yoga began thousands of years ago with the first yoga practitioner who sat on a blanket instead of in the dirt. Or with the first yogis to use a strap to support their legs so they could sit longer in meditation. (This is actually the earliest example of the use of yoga props from more than two thousand years ago.[3]) But the idea of adapting the pose to the person, instead of the person to the pose, is a relatively new one.

Only recently has there started to be some serious questioning about what's really happening in yoga on many levels: culturally, psychologically, and physiologically.[4] This questioning is shifting the focus more to the individual's experience and intuition, and to a deeper understanding of the practice.

Unfortunately, modern postural yoga has stumbled many times. There has been an unacceptable amount of abuse and injury. Now we need to find a new way to approach the practice. The goal of Accessible Yoga is to find an inclusive and equitable practice that is safe and effective and still respectful of the Indian roots of yoga.

The fall of traditional Indian gurus led to the rise of a Westernized practice that reeks of colonization and commercialization. As yoga becomes more intertwined with capitalism, the yoga community must grapple with many questions, including: Who has the right to the teachings and practices of yoga? Is yoga reserved only for people with a certain body type? Is yoga mainly a physical practice of putting the body in various prescribed poses? How can we practice in a way that is in alignment with the long tradition of yoga?

By shifting our understanding of yoga away from the perfect images we see in magazines or on social media, we can expand our perception of yoga and how it can serve the diversity of humankind. Like light through a prism, Accessible Yoga expands the teachings of yoga to expose their endless variations and applications.

In this book, I'll explore the practice of yoga for real people with real, diverse bodies rather than start with the idea of yoga as a set of physical practices that we should all aspire to do and that can only be performed by people who we should aspire to look like. I'm starting with a different idea: we are all valuable and equally deserving of yoga. It is not just for a select few, but for *every body*.

This book is not meant to be prescriptive in any way. In fact, I'm particularly interested in approaching the practices of yoga with a creative spirit and a fresh eye. Think of each practice as a different paint color and each day is an opportunity to paint a new picture that expresses how you feel in this moment in a personal and profound way. And just like with any creative endeavor, this is only possible when you let go of preconceived ideas of how yoga is supposed to be done or how it's supposed to look. Instead, I hope you'll consider the role of each practice and what it's designed to do. With this understanding, you can create a personal yoga practice that is designed just for you.

To help with this process, I'll introduce you to Accessible Yoga practitioners who have found creative and original ways to adapt yoga for themselves and who exemplify the creative spirit of yoga. Through their example, you'll gain insight into the process of personalizing a yoga practice and learn about different options and possibilities.

Throughout the book I'll offer short practices so you can stop and experience the concept that I'm trying to teach. I'll end with outlines of some sample classes you can do on your own, which you can use as a springboard for the exploration of your body and mind. But first, let go of your preconceived ideas about what yoga is: yoga is not about having a flexible body; it's about having a flexible mind, and it's accessible to all of us.

PART ONE

MAKING YOGA ACCESSIBLE

ACCESSIBLE YOGA PHILOSOPHY 1

I REALIZE this chapter title can have two meanings: making the philosophy of yoga accessible and understanding the philosophy of Accessible Yoga as a movement and a nonprofit organization. Hopefully those two things are basically the same. Let's explore both. The accessible yoga movement has been going on longer than the Accessible Yoga organization has been around. As an organization, we are simply voicing what so many yoga practitioners have been saying for years—that yoga belongs to all of us! You can consider the mission statement for Accessible Yoga, the nonprofit, to get a clear idea of what we're trying to do.

> **Accessible Yoga Mission Statement**
>
> Accessible Yoga is dedicated to sharing the benefits of yoga with anyone who currently does not have access to these practices, and with communities that have been excluded or underserved. All people, regardless of ability or background, deserve equal access to the ancient practices of yoga, which offer individual empowerment and spiritual awakening.
>
> By building a strong network and advocating for a diverse yoga culture that is inclusive and welcoming, we are sharing yoga with all.

The nonprofit organization grew out of the classes I was teaching for people with disabilities. I was simultaneously leading yoga teacher training programs and kept trying to encourage my students with disabilities to attend them and become yoga teachers. But most of the students felt that the trainings weren't accessible. So, in 2007, I created a basic yoga teacher training for people with disabilities to become yoga teachers under the name Accessible Yoga.

I also started offering Accessible Yoga Trainings so teachers could learn how to make their teaching accessible. Finally, the Accessible Yoga Conferences arose because I found myself searching for support for this work, and I couldn't find any. After years of frustration, I finally decided to create what I was searching for and to focus my energy on supporting all the yoga teachers and practitioners who shared the vision of yoga for all.

Now let's consider what it means to make yoga philosophy accessible. The word *philosophy* can be off-putting, but please don't be afraid to read and study yoga philosophy and the amazing texts where the teachings are found. Going directly to the source is very powerful, and in the case of yoga, the sources are accessible.

There are literally hundreds of translations of the Yoga Sutras of Patanjali and the Bhagavad Gita, the two main historical texts of yoga. If possible, don't read just one translation; find a few different versions that inspire you and make you think. Some translations are very academic, but others are more easily understandable. If one version doesn't work for you, find another.

You don't need to read them straight through like a book. Instead, explore a section at a time and consider how to apply the ideas in your yoga practice. This could mean using concepts from the texts in your meditation or throughout your day. We'll explore what a yoga practice means in the next chapter.

The teachings shared in these texts create a context for our own exploration of yoga. It connects us to yoga practitioners over the ages and helps us understand what yoga is. Personally, when I do something, I always ask myself, "Why am I doing this?" and, "Is this supporting me in making a positive change in my life and positive change in the world?" These questions are essential for any spiritual practice.

The paradox of yoga is that it's simultaneously personal and communal, individual and universal. We go in and out. We turn within for inner connection, then we reach out to connect with others. Yoga teaches me that my destiny is wound up in the destiny of all other beings. As much as I might feel that I am an isolated island, I'm really just a wave in this immense human ocean.

YOGA AND HUMAN RIGHTS

I imagine that for most people talking about yoga and human rights in the same sentence may seem strange. But this connection became clear in my mind when I had the privilege of attending a special event at the United

Nations (UN) Human Rights Commission in Geneva in 2015. The event was the celebration of the International Day of Persons with Disabilities, December 3, a holiday established by the UN. That year, I was invited to teach Accessible Yoga as part of a variety of offerings focusing on the positive steps that people with disabilities can take to achieve full equality and enjoy basic human rights.

Most of the other presenters were leaders of disability rights groups from around the globe. They spoke about how people with disabilities make up the largest minority group in the world—well over one billion people! And they discussed the basic human rights that they are seeking for people with disabilities.

In 2006, the UN's Human Rights Commission set the gold standard for these human rights in its Convention on the Rights of Persons with Disabilities. The commission declared, "The purpose of the present Convention is to promote, protect and ensure the full and equal enjoyment of all human rights and fundamental freedoms by all persons with disabilities, and to promote respect for their inherent dignity."[1]

I was struck by the correlation between basic human rights and the fundamental teachings of yoga philosophy. According to the yoga tradition, each person has a spiritual essence, which is called the *atman*, or *purusha*. The work of yoga (the poses, breathing practices, ethical living, and meditation) are all about opening the pathways to remember that essence. I've always loved the fact that yoga begins with this positive assumption.

The idea is that every single one of us has an atman, and that there is no differentiation made between the atman of any two people, regardless of their ability or background. Yoga begins with equality, as we are all equal in spirit. And because we are all equal in spirit, yoga has equal potential for helping anyone, of any background or ability, to find the inner peace that we all crave.

Of course, embracing diversity is an essential part of human rights, and the disability community is extremely diverse. There is currently a shift in the disability community toward disability pride, toward embracing difference. As a gay man, pride has a special meaning to me. I grew up thinking that being gay was a deficit. I have learned to be proud of my differences, and this shift has been a great source of my healing. Now I am not only proud of being gay, but I see how being different makes me stronger.

Swami Sivananda, my teacher's teacher, used to say that spiritual life is about seeing the "unity in diversity." This means being able to see that we are all connected and simultaneously to embrace our differences. Yoga and human rights both stem from this dual vision—the ability to hold both equality and diversity simultaneously. It's really a paradox: we are all the same and yet all unique.

This perspective is challenging in a modern world where some people are empowered and some are not, a world that is filled with division and the separation of groups based on race, class, gender identity, political affiliation, and so on. Our job as yoga practitioners and human rights advocates is to embrace those differences and at the same time to see the same essence in everyone we meet.

According to the Bhagavad Gita (6.29–32), as we become more in tune with ourselves, we begin to experience that underlying connection with others. Krishna, who is teaching Arjuna how to be a yogi, explains,

> As your mind becomes harmonized through yoga practices, you begin to see the Atman in all beings and all beings in your Self; you see the same Self everywhere and in everything. Those who see me wherever they look and recognize everything as my manifestation, never again feel separate from me, nor I from them. Whoever becomes established in the all-pervading oneness and worships me abiding in all beings—however he may be living, that yogi lives in me. The yogi who perceives the essential oneness everywhere naturally feels the pleasure or pain of others as his or her own.[2]

Amazingly, Krishna is saying that seeing through the diversity of nature to experience the oneness of creation isn't enough. He is teaching us that once we go down that path, we will literally feel the pleasure and pain of others as our own. That's the ultimate level of awareness—true connection. And that is the first step on the path to equality and human rights. If we feel intimately connected to others, then we automatically take care of them.

But this can only happen if we understand our personal privilege and the perspective we are coming from; otherwise that concept of oneness can be used to avoid the harsh reality of human rights abuse and leave us complacent. This is called spiritual bypassing, as explained by Michelle Cassandra Johnson:

> Spiritual bypassing perpetuates the idea that the belief "we are one" is enough to create a reality where we are treated equally and as one. It is not. Spiritual bypassing permits the status quo to stay in place and teaches people that if you believe in something and have a good intent that is enough. It is not.[3]

This paradox of unity and diversity is at the heart of yoga and at the heart of human rights. With practice, self-awareness, and action, we can deepen our experience of yoga, reconnecting with our essence and simultaneously begin to address human rights and discrimination honestly and openly. The form this takes in the world is service, or karma yoga.

Some shocking recent research shows that yoga and meditation practice can actually build the ego—the opposite of what we might expect.[4] This may be because yoga can increase our energy and support whatever is already in our minds. Without a focus on service, this increased energy may simply support our general self-centered approach to life. Without service, spiritual power is simply power.

On the other hand, service is spiritual practice in action. Service means that we solidify that spiritual experience in the world. It offers us a way to make the heart-opening, third-eye-opening process of transformation into something real and useful in the world. It's essential to find a form for your service; otherwise spiritual practice is ineffective. It's not so much about "helping" others; it's about helping yourself and truly seeing yourself in others.

Some people serve naturally as an expression of the way they are in the world; others come by service other ways. When my husband and I adopted our kids, I had no idea what I was in for. I remember when they were infants, getting up many times during the night to feed them, change them, do whatever was needed. I never had to stop and ask, "What's in it for me?" My love for them moved me to serve them without question. It was an amazing (and exhausting) experience.

People who are serving tirelessly—parents, caregivers, anyone in the service professions—need to work on self-care so that they have more energy for their service. One of the challenges for people who are caring for others is learning how much to care for themselves. There's a precarious balance between service and self-care, and one of the most important things we can do as yoga practitioners is find that balance.

✖ Try It: Self-Care and Service

Sit comfortably and take a few breaths. Reflect on the following questions. Note your responses and come back to them later.

- What are some ways that I practice self-care?
- What are some ways that I offer service in the world? (Note that service is not the same as volunteering. You can serve your loved ones, your garden, your friends, and so on.)

- Is there a way that I can integrate my self-care and my service? Or is there a way to balance them in my life?
- Notice what answers come, or journal about them.

. . . . ⁚⁚

CALM THE MIND

If you ask most people what yoga is, they'll tell you it's either a bunch of funny poses with animal names or advanced gymnastics that most people could never do. I wonder how many people would answer that yoga is about calming the mind to connect with love in the heart? The Yoga Sutras of Patanjali is considered to be one of the main sources of the yoga teachings from about fifteen hundred years ago. It contains 196 short verses called *sutras* in Sanskrit, the ancient language of yoga.

The second sutra is often quoted as the definition of yoga, *yogas chitta vritti nirodhah*. It can be translated as, "Yoga is the stilling of the turnings of the mind."[5] But I like to think of it in more accessible terms: calm the mind, free the heart. In fact, here's my personal take on some of the most essential sutras in the first chapter of the Yoga Sutras of Patanjali:

1.1 We're doing yoga now (stop texting).

1.2 Calm the mind, free the heart.

1.3 Then you know you're home.

1.4 Otherwise you're lost in the endless worry, fear, and anxiety of life.

1.5 Sometimes you feel relaxed and sometimes stressed, but in the end you need to go deeper to find the truth.

1.6 Your mind is either right or wrong, or you're just making stuff up. What is real? You like to sleep and live in the past, but neither one holds the answer.

1.12 If you really want to understand, then do your practice and release your grip on the world.

1.13 Doing yoga means paying attention . . .

1.14 . . . for a long time, not just a couple of minutes. You have to really want it.

1.15 In the end, letting go and loving is always the answer.

1.16 Really.

Before we can calm our minds and free our hearts, we need to start by bringing awareness to our inner dialogue, which is called *svadhaya*. So much can be learned through this kind of self-reflection. According to the yoga teachings, there is an awareness or universal consciousness that's always there, silently watching as the mind goes through its ups and downs.

This awareness was there when you were a child, a teen, an adult, and as you age—the part of you that doesn't change even though the body and the mind are changing. This part even continues after you die. In many ways, the goal of yoga is to get the mind quiet enough to expose or reveal the unchanging awareness that is always there.

As you become more aware of the inner dialogue, you can begin to listen more closely to the voice, or voices, in your head. You're always talking to yourself, aren't you? The real question is, who is talking and who is listening? If your mind is talking and the universal consciousness within you is listening, is that some kind of prayer? Perhaps you're praying all day long and you don't realize it!

The mind is in endless dialogue (prayer) with the universal consciousness within. You have that silent witness listening to all your hopes and dreams. Maybe with increased awareness you can be a little more thoughtful about what you're praying for. Have you heard the expression, "Worry is praying for what you don't want to happen"?

Through the process of reflection, you can begin to hear the voices that aren't yours—internalized voices. Some of these voices might be positive or neutral, like a loving parent or friend. Or they might be negative and critical. When you make a mistake, what do you say to yourself? Do you say, "You're so stupid"? Or do you say, "You're doing your best"?

Occasionally, I notice my own internalized homophobia saying things that I would never say out loud to anyone! This kind of internalized oppression is especially harmful for those of us who struggle with external oppression such as ableism, racism, sexism, transphobia, and so forth. The question is, can we use the tools of yoga and meditation to slowly heal those wounds?

⠶ Try It: Talking to Myself Meditation ·······················

Sit comfortably. Take a few full breaths and notice the effects of deep breathing.

- Begin to observe your mind without trying to stop the thoughts.
- Become extra observant of your inner dialogue; listen to the tone of voice and feeling behind the thoughts.
- As your mind talks, listen to it carefully, because what we all need is a really good listener.
- Listen attentively to your own mind. Hear the thoughts.

- See if you can listen to the thoughts without getting involved in their stories.
- Who is talking?
- Who is listening?
- After a few minutes of listening to your mind, take a few full breaths with extended exhalations and open your eyes.
- Notice how you feel.

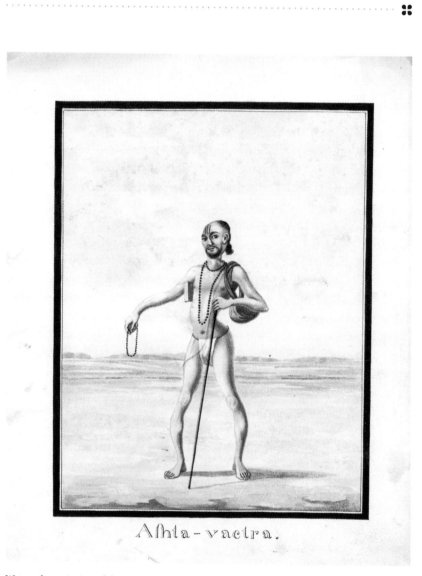

Aſhta-vactra.

Watercolor painting of the yogic sage Ashtavakra, by an anonymous artist, Patna District of India, early 19th century. © The Trustees of the British Museum. All rights reserved.

FREE THE HEART

A revered figure in the yoga tradition is the sage Ashtavakra, whose name literally means "eight bends." He may have lived more than three thousand years ago in India, although his exact history is unclear. There is even a complicated yoga pose (Ashtavakrasana, which is a side Crow Pose) named after him, which I won't be covering in this book!

The story of Ashtavakra began when he was a fetus in his mother's womb, listening to his father reciting the Vedas, the most ancient Indian teachings. From the womb, Ashtavakra corrected his father's pronunciation. Furious at this criticism from his unborn son, Ashtavakra's father attempted to curse him with eight bends in his body.

This is a great moment to consider ableism and the idea that having a disability is a curse. *Ableism* is discrimination based on disability and the misunderstanding that there is an ideal "normal" way to be in the world. Ableism is particularly insidious because it can lead to dehumanizing and extreme reactions. Often people with disabilities are seen as either subhuman or superhuman, when neither is the case. We are all simply human, with our strengths and weaknesses. To overcome ableism, we need to normalize different bodies and abilities as an integrated part of the human experience.

Of course, Ashtavakra's story is part of yoga's mythology so it tends toward hyperbole. He went on to become a very important teacher in the yoga tradition, and I'm sure his experience having a disability was an important part of his wisdom. He was a masterful teacher who could see beyond the limitations of the physical body, and his teachings were powerful spiritual revelations.

Ashtavakra was also able to see beyond the limitations of class and position. In another famous story, King Janaka became a disciple of Ashtavakra's and began to study at his ashram. This was shocking to everyone in the kingdom because normally a king is interested only in materialism and not in spirituality. The other monks at the ashram were shocked when Ashtavakra accepted King Janaka as his student, and they felt that Ashtavakra was being corrupted by the king and his wealth.

In response, Ashtavakra found a way to teach his students about nonattachment (freedom from selfish desire). He designed a test for them. He had one of his aides run into the ashram during meditation and yell, "Fire, fire, the whole kingdom is on fire!" Hearing this, the monks all jumped up out of meditation and ran to check on their huts to see if their meager belongings were safe from the fire. But all during this commotion, King Janaka remained deep in meditation, completely undisturbed. He was so focused on his spiritual practice that he proved he wasn't attached to worldly possessions, which in his case included the entire kingdom.

This story touches on an important aspect of nonattachment—healing our relationship to the people and things in our lives. As you begin to listen to your inner dialogue, you might notice how much of that chatter is related to what you want or, perhaps even more, what you don't want to happen. Attachment and its opposite, aversion, are the content of most of our thoughts. It is only by finding a path through the thicket of these thoughts that we find peace. Ashtavakra speaks directly to this point in the Ashtavakra Gita (1.1–1.4, 1.11):

1. O Master,
   Tell me how to find
   Detachment, wisdom, and freedom!

2. Child,
   If you wish to be free,
   Shun the poison of the senses.

   Seek the nectar of truth,
   Of love and forgiveness,
   Simplicity and happiness.

3. Earth, fire and water,
   The wind and the sky—
   You are none of these.

   If you wish to be free,
   Know you are the Self,
   The witness of all these,
   The heart of awareness.

4. Set your body aside.
   Sit in your own awareness.

   You will at once be happy,
   Forever still,
   Forever free.

   . . . .

11. If you think you are free,
    You are free.

    If you think you are bound,
    You are bound.

    For the saying is true:
    You are what you think.[6]

Ashtavakra's teachings are found in the Ashtavakra Gita (although it's unclear if he actually wrote this text). The Ashtavakra Gita echoes many themes from the Yoga Sutras of Patanjali, which the writer was probably familiar with. In both texts, we are offered a variety of different ways to work with the mind and find freedom. These include yoga practices you may have already heard about, such as breathing practices and meditation. There are also many incredibly useful yoga tools that you don't hear much about, such as nonattachment, which in Sanskrit is *vairagya*. (Note: Vairagya has nothing to do with Viagra. In fact, they may have opposite meanings—dispassion versus passion!)

Basically, an attachment is something outside yourself that you think you need in order to be happy. Thoughts like, "If this relationship were better, then I'd be happy," or "If I made more money, then I'd be happy," or "When I'm healthy, then I'll be happy." But living between the "if" and "then" is claustrophobic. There's no room in that space to honestly explore who you are. Even worse, it represents a misunderstanding about how to be happy.

According to yoga, happiness is an inside job. Sure, you may get a momentary high from getting something you desire, but you'll also be depressed when that thing is taken away. According to the yoga teachings, lasting happiness comes through peace of mind, through contentment. Peace comes through nonattachment. This is contrary to the Western mind-set that the fulfillment of desire brings happiness.

In the Yoga Sutras (2.42), Patanjali teaches us that contentment, nonattachment, is the key to happiness. He even explains, "By contentment supreme joy is gained."[7] Do you agree? Aren't we taught that joy and happiness come through the achievement of our goals? How is it that contentment, a form of gratitude for what we currently have, can bring supreme joy? In many ways, this is a transformational idea and a key secret of yoga.

Perhaps it's the secret of yoga because it is the ultimate form of empowerment. Nonattachment offers you the power to choose peace of mind even if the external situation is not what you want it to be. As Ashtavakra teaches us, "If you think you are free, you are free. If you think you are bound, you are bound."

Nonattachment is an essential part of coming to grips with aging, illness, and death. Sometimes the vision of what our lives are supposed to look like can interfere with enjoying the lives we are actually living. The fact is, we're all dying, and most of us will get sick along the way. At some point we have to face that whatever idealized vision we have for our future will eventually crumble, because everything in the physical world is impermanent. Even as you read that, notice what feelings come up for you. Do you want to avoid thinking about it, or are you at peace with that idea?

The goal of nonattachment is to connect with a deeper aspect of ourselves rather than grasping on to things that are constantly changing. With an illness or a disability, the experience of that condition can change day to day, hour to hour. There is no one way to be sick, just as there is no one way to be healthy. In fact, what does "being healthy" really mean? Can you have an illness or a disability and be healthy, whole, and complete? Can you be healed in a deeper way? Can you even be healed and die? Or is death some kind of failure of healing? Here is a meditation to help you expand your concept of healing.

⁘ Try It: What Is Healing? Meditation

Take a moment to get comfortable physically and mentally. Take a few breaths and allow your mind to focus.

Ask yourself these questions. (If it's useful, write the answers in a journal.)

- What does healing mean to me?
- Can I have a problem, an illness, or a disability and still be healed?
- How do I feel about getting older?
- How do I feel about dying?
- What do I need to discover within myself in order to experience healing?

Spend some time in reflection on these questions. Write down your thoughts and then leave them for a day or two. Come back later and see if they resonate with you.

This always makes me think of the deep lesson in nonattachment that my best friend, Kurt, taught me as he was dying of AIDS. He was passionate about philosophy and had studied all kinds of spiritual traditions. Through his study, he felt that the concept of nonattachment summarized all the spiritual lessons that we need to learn—basically, how to let go.

Kurt was a writer, and he loved to make lists. Whenever we were hanging out, he would pass the time by making lists of things like "All the people I'd ever dated" or "My favorite foods." As Kurt got sicker, it became clear that his medical treatment was failing, and he only had a short time to live. Amazingly, he thought of combining his passion for making lists with his desire to work on releasing his attachments, saying good-bye to all the things he loved as he was consciously dying. So he decided to make a list of his attachments every day, and as he wrote them out, he would try to say good-bye to each one.

After a few weeks of doing this practice every day, Kurt told me that he had gotten his list of attachments down to four things:

1. His partner, Randy
2. His dog, Buddy
3. His apartment
4. Me, his best friend (I was excited to make the top four!)

Then Kurt got a lot sicker. He had lymphoma, which made his face swell so much that he was unrecognizable; Kaposi's sarcoma, dark lesions all over his skin; and retinitis, which was making him go blind. He ended up in the hospital, and one day when I went to see him, I noticed he was in a really good mood. I asked, "Why are you in such a good mood? Aren't you supposed to be depressed when you're so sick and in the hospital?" He said, "I got my list of attachments down to only two!"

1. Randy
2. Buddy

I was kind of shocked. I said, "Wait. I'm off the list? How is that a good thing?" He then took the opportunity to say good-bye to me and explain about nonattachment. "Yes" he said, "you're my dear spiritual friend. I love you, and we'll always be together."

At that moment I didn't really comprehend the magnitude of what he was saying to me, but later after he died, I realized that he had given me a great gift. Kurt had consciously said good-bye to me and shown me the power of nonattachment: freedom from the mind's wants and desires. It is freedom from a cage that we construct for ourselves.

⁝ *Try It: Practicing Nonattachment* ···································

Take a moment to close your eyes and center yourself.

Notice sensations in your body. For example, notice the solidness of the floor or chair or bed beneath you, the temperature of the air, or any sounds you may hear.

Bring your awareness to the breath.

Ask yourself these questions.

- What is bothering me right now?
- Am I suffering in some way?
- If so, can I clearly identify what is causing that suffering?
- Do I have an attachment that is at the root of this suffering? (Remember, an attachment is something in the outside world we're basing our happiness on.)
- What is the attachment?
- Can I imagine letting it go?
- How would that feel?

Sit for a few minutes exploring the feeling of letting go of the attachment. It's important to note that you can still have that thing in your life, even if you release your attachment to it. Releasing it allows you to feel at peace with or without the object of attachment. Take a deep breath and acknowledge how you feel.

··· ⁝

A REVOLUTIONARY PRACTICE   2

yuvā vṛddho 'tivṛddho vā vyādhito durbalo 'pi vā |
abhyāsāt siddhim āpnoti sarvayogeṣv atandritaḥ ||
Haṭhapradīpikā 1.64

Whether young, old, very old, diseased, or weak, one who
practices untiringly attains success in all yogas.
—Hatha Yoga Pradipika, Yogi Swatmarama[1]
(fifteenth century C.E.)

LET'S FACE IT, extreme flexibility isn't much of an accomplishment. In fact, flexibility in conditions like Ehlers-Danlos syndrome and hypermobility joint syndrome can be a dangerous thing. In these cases, you may be too flexible and need to work on finding more stability and strength to protect your joints. Recently, there have been reports of avid yoga practitioners getting hip replacements at a young age, in part because of a yoga practice that continually takes the joints outside of the normal range of motion.[2]

Modern postural yoga has become an extreme sport. It has chosen to value, and even fetishize, the gymnastic side of yoga rather than a balanced practice that is safe and effective. Maybe it's because subtle, gentle movements don't look as dramatic in advertising campaigns selling yoga clothing or on social media. Maybe it's because of our competitive nature, which teaches us that more is always better, even when it's not.

I've been training yoga teachers for more than twenty years, and I come across a lot of confusion and misunderstanding about what yoga is about and how to practice safely. Invariably, when I'm training teachers how to adapt yoga for students with disabilities or limited mobility, someone will ask, "What about the integrity of the pose? Don't you lose something when you adapt the practice?" This is in reference to the idea that if you modify these classic poses, you end up with something less than yoga. My answer to this question is always, "People are more important than poses, and it's better to adapt a pose to a person than a person to a pose."

You could say that each yoga pose is like a question, and each person has a slightly different answer to that question. No answer is wrong or right. They're all unique. Plus, we're all changing moment to moment, and what is right for us one day may be wrong the next. I always suggest finding the essence of a pose by asking yourself why you are doing it. You can explore this through practice and study. With that deeper understanding, it becomes possible to adapt your practice to a personal and creative expression of your spirit.

Yoga scholars are talking about how we're moving into a time of "post-lineage yoga."[3] This is a time when we gather together in yoga studios, community centers, conferences, festivals, and even online to find our *sangha*, or spiritual community. It's no longer common to be practicing in ashrams with a guru, and many gurus have been shown to be abusive in some way. Instead, we are finding a new format for the practice as yoga continues to grow and expand.

When you look at yoga history, you find that there really isn't just one straightforward narrative. It's an ancient and complex tapestry of traditions woven together into this thing that we refer to as yoga. It's always adapting and growing according to time and place.

Yoga's history is punctuated by great teachers, or gurus. These gurus were masterful teachers who innovated yoga in some way. Most of them took the practice that they were taught and used their own creativity to make something new.

Creativity is the heart of spirituality and the heart of yoga. When we simply copy what we're taught, our practice can become stagnant and ineffective. You can think of the gurus like famous painters. If you want to be a painter, then copying famous paintings can only get you so far. It is a great way to learn about painting. But, at some point, you need to express your own creativity, take the tools you learn and find your own way.

Also, it's interesting to note how important community is in the practice of yoga. We need the support of like-minded people to keep our practice alive. I encourage you to find or create your own sangha. Practicing alone with this book is a great start, but eventually yoga needs to be shared. Our personal healing is woven into the healing of our family, our friends, and our community. Can you use this book to help you create a yoga community? Perhaps you can practice with a friend or family member. Maybe it will inspire you to attend a group yoga class. Or even to become a yoga teacher and create the kind of community that you are seeking.

Why Practice?

In his Yoga Sutras, Patanjali defines yoga practice as "effort toward steadiness of mind" (1:13).[4] This is an important concept to remember because it's so easy to get caught up in the idea that yoga is about making complicated shapes with your body. The idea that yoga practice is about steadying the mind logically follows Patanjali's earlier challenge: calm the mind, free the heart.

To me, this not only seems like a much loftier goal than contorting my body like a pretzel but a much more valuable one. So much of the time my mind seems to have a mind of its own! Like those nights when I'm lying in bed and my mind won't stop obsessing over some mean comment someone made to me in passing. Or when I try to meditate and my mind feels more like a runaway train than a peaceful lotus blossom.

Recently, I've been reflecting on why my mind is so busy all the time. What does all that activity achieve? If I'm being honest, I think it's about avoiding uncomfortable or painful feelings—anything from disappointment to dismay, boredom to frustration. My mind would rather scroll through my Facebook feed (again) than feel those feelings.

In the end, the energy from those emotions gets stuck in my body, unfelt, like layers of sediment getting compressed into rock. Practice is like an archaeological dig, and asana is my shovel. Sometimes what I discover under all those painful layers is joy, like a hidden diamond. Those diamond moments occur when I'm practicing yoga and I feel present and connected to myself. Practice is making the effort to bring my awareness back to my heart—to free my heart—even if it's uneasy or painful.

As a parent, partner, teacher, business owner, and friend, I often put other people's needs before my own. Sometimes creating space for my yoga practice feels selfish and at odds with my dedication to loving and serving those around me. But as I get older and practice more, I see that these two things are not mutually exclusive. In fact, the way I take care of other people is by taking care of myself.

Is it selfish to take fifteen minutes, or even an hour, every day to practice yoga? Or can your practice nourish you so that you're better able to serve those around you? Can it give you strength, self-awareness, and kindness when they're most needed?

I'm reminded of a story my friend once told me about how her yoga practice helps her. She said that one day she was standing at her kitchen window and saw a bad car accident on the street in front of her house. Her neighbor across the street ran out and stood in the middle of the street screaming and crying. Instead of joining in the chaos, my friend calmly picked up the phone and called 911. She said that her ability to stay calm enough to call for help was a direct result of her practice and a great example of how her practice and the centeredness that she found served other people.

Taken one step further, consider how revolutionary it is for those of us who are struggling with sexism, racism, homophobia, transphobia, ableism, or any kind of oppression to care for ourselves. The act of self-care becomes an act of defiance to a culture that is built on disempowerment because it gives us back our power.

One of the ultimate acts of power is discovering our own happiness and peace of mind without relying on external circumstances. Yoga practice is the ideal self-care practice because it is based on the premise that we have what we need inside and that happiness arises through contentment rather than through achievement or accumulation of possessions.

How to Practice

There are so many benefits to yoga—some have been proven by medical research, and some we hear about through the intuitive experience of practitioners. There are also many great resources with more information on the benefits of yoga, which I encourage you to find. That is particularly important if you're looking to use yoga to care for a specific condition or illness. You can refer to the "Resources" section at the back of this book as a starting point.

Among other things, yoga has been shown to help the body's inflammatory response (through toning the vagus nerve[5]), as well as reverse heart disease[6] and improve brain health.[7] Yoga has also been shown to improve depression and anxiety,[8] as well as support our general physical and mental health. But yoga's most important benefit may be in making us more resilient to stress,[9] which is associated with so many health conditions and is such a major issue in contemporary society.

Sometimes we read about these kinds of medical benefits and think that we just need more yoga and we'll be cured of whatever ails us. It's important to remember that movement and meditation are powerful additions to your health care regimen, which should also include other kinds of exercise, regular medical care, psychological support, and community. Yoga is not intended to replace quality health care.

So what is it about moving your body into shapes that offers so much benefit, quiets your mind, and makes you feel grounded and present? Yoga poses grab your attention through sensation and movement. That is why you need to focus your mind to make your asana practice most effective.

Begin by focusing on any sensations that you're feeling, physically and emotionally. For example, the stability of the ground beneath you, where you feel a stretch or release in your body, or where you encounter resistance or discomfort. This is how you can practice safely, by being aware of how you're feeling and noticing if you're straining or having any pain. In that case, it's best to ease up or come out of a pose.

It's important to find the point in a pose where there is a little bit of a challenge to your body but you're not straining. Once you're straining, you may start losing some of the health benefits of the practice, such as reducing inflammation and stress. Sometimes this means limiting the amount of movement or stretch in a pose, and sometimes it means coming out of the pose completely.

I don't offer specific timing for any practices in this book. I am leaving this open on purpose for your own exploration. If you're a beginner, then take it easy. Only spend a few breaths in a pose, or try coming in and out of the pose a few times to notice how it feels. After a few weeks of practicing, you can begin to spend a little more time in the pose.

Some disabilities interfere with your ability to sense when you've pushed too far. In that case you'll need to explore different ways to sense when you're overdoing it in your practice. Sometimes you won't be able to tell until later. Do you have more or less pain the next day? If you have more, then you may have gone too far.

The breath is also a particularly effective focus for your mind because your breath is always in the present moment. You can't breathe in the future or in the past, can you? Similarly, peace of mind can only be experienced in the present moment. All the planning in the world doesn't create peace of mind. Present moment awareness does. Also, if you're straining, the breath may quicken, or you may feel out of breath. This is a signal that you should slow down or ease up on the practice.

Here are a few different ways to focus the mind during practice. I recommend beginning with the first ones and experimenting with the others over time. Also, as we look at the poses in the next sections, we'll consider specific areas to focus on in each pose.

1. General sensations in the body/energy moving
2. Breath
3. The connection between the breath and movement
4. A specific internal point in the body (for example, the heart center or third eye)
5. An external point outside the body (helpful for balancing poses)

Yoga is intended to increase interoception, or awareness of our inner world. This is a powerful benefit as it can allow us to become more sensitive to what's happening to us physically and psychologically. It's important to trust this inner sense and not always think more is better. If you're feeling pain in a yoga pose, come out of it. If you find that meditation is bringing up painful feelings, stop doing it. Trust your instincts, and reach out for help if you need it.

Sometimes previous trauma can be released during practice, and you may feel emotional. It's important to get support to handle these feelings and not continually push yourself harder and further. In other words, the most useful yoga practice is one that is in balance with the rest of your life, a practice that makes you feel a little calmer and more connected with your body.

FINDING THE ESSENCE OF A POSE

Asana (the Sanskrit word for yoga pose) is just one part of yoga, but it's an important part, and it can be made accessible to everyone who is interested. The question everyone has is, "How do I start? How do I find a way into a practice that seems so physically challenging?" The answer is to start where you are.

When you consider practicing a new yoga pose, it's easy to look at the "full expression" of the pose and think, "I'll never be able to do that." The fact is, the full expression of a pose—or an advanced variation—isn't actually better than any other variation. Remember, peace of mind is the goal of yoga, and physical ability does *not* correlate to peace of mind. Someone who is strong and flexible is not necessarily more peaceful.

To practice yoga, we need to understand the relationship between its physical practices and the subtle practices such as relaxation, breathing, and meditation. In fact, in yoga, more subtle is more powerful. Asana practice creates an opportunity for the mind to get quiet, but your ability to quiet your mind is not the result of how "advanced" the pose you're doing is; it's actually the result of how focused you are. It's not what you do, but how you do it.

My first yoga teacher, Kazuko, also happened to be a master of the Japanese tea ceremony. She showed me how the seemingly simple act of making a cup of tea can be turned into an art form and a spiritual practice. It wasn't the complexity or difficulty of making the tea that made it special. On the contrary, it was the simplicity of the practice and the ability to stay completely focused in the present moment that was key. The same is true in yoga.

This present moment awareness can also help us find that balance between stretching and straining in our practice. Pushing too hard in asana and practicing variations that are too advanced can move us away from the goal of yoga. Similarly, giving up and thinking, "I'll never be able to do that pose" misses the point.

For example, think of Cobra Pose (Bhujangasana), where you lie face-down on the ground and raise your head, neck, and chest. If you look at images of Cobra Pose on social media, you'll probably think, "Forget it!" This is a shame because it is one of the poses that offers benefit for almost everyone.

So what can you do? If you can't get down on the floor, does that mean you can't practice Cobra Pose? No, because there are endless variations of this asana, including practicing in a chair, kneeling, standing, or lying in bed. In fact, there are as many variations of Cobra Pose as there are people practicing it.

So the way to start practicing a new pose is to consider, "Why do this practice, and what are the benefits?" Cobra Pose has many benefits, but let's focus on two main ones. It is great for posture, since it strengthens the upper back and moves the spine in the opposite direction of our normal slouching position. It is also a heart-opener, which means it expands the area of the chest around the heart and allows us to expose our emotional heart to the world.

⠶ *Try It: Creating Cobra Pose*

First, think of the energetic movements of Cobra Pose, including expanding the chest and strengthening the upper back. How can you create the experience of the pose where you are right now?

- Begin by trying to experience Cobra Pose in your mind.
- Imagine lengthening your spine and creating a gentle arch in your upper back and neck.
- Then see if you can experience it in a very gentle way in your body by slowly moving into that shape and expanding the area around your heart. These can be micromovements that are barely visible to the eye.
- Notice all the sensations you experience in your body; notice what your breath is doing.
- Then rest and notice how you feel after practicing that pose.
- The moment after you do a practice is very important. Always take a moment after each pose to notice how you feel: what changed physically, emotionally, and mentally?

Props Can Create Alignment

Alignment is the most overused word in asana practice. There really isn't much agreement about what the perfect alignment should be in any given pose. Instead, I like to think of alignment as "practicing safely." That means that alignment is different for each person in each situation. Props can keep you safe by allowing your body to remain in alignment as you practice, which can prevent you from overstretching or straining parts of your body.

⁑ *Try It: Use a Strap in Seated Forward Bend*

If you're able to get down to the floor, try practicing a seated forward bend. Or you can practice in a chair.

- *From a mat:* Start by sitting with both legs stretched out in front of you.
- Bend your left leg, take your knee out to the side, and place the sole of your left foot against your right inner thigh.
- *From a chair:* Sit tall and stretch your right leg out in front of you without holding it.
- *From a chair or mat:* Keep your right leg extended in front of you, and slowly reach your hands toward your right foot, without straining.
- Notice if you're rounding your back as you begin to reach toward your toes. That rounding in your low back (spinal flexion) can cause strain and potential injury.
- Now try placing a strap around the ball of your right foot, holding the two ends of the strap with your hands and giving yourself as much slack as you need so that you can keep your spine long and your back tall.

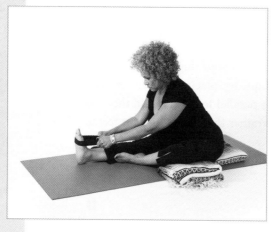
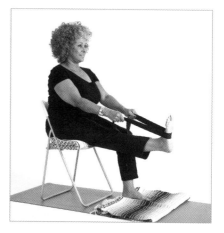

- Inhale, lengthen your spine, and try hinging gently forward at your hips (hip flexion). This is a much safer position and provides better alignment for your spine as opposed to rounding your lower back (spinal flexion).

Props Help Make Connections

Many of the benefits of asana practice have to do with the flow of energy (*prana*) within you as you open and relax your body. In asana practice we often find important connections between parts of our bodies, or our bodies and the floor, that encourage this energy flow. Like mudras (gestures) that allow energy to move and expand, each asana allows energy to move and open in a certain way. You can use props to connect parts of your body that may not otherwise connect and to close the circuit, increasing the feeling of energy flowing through your body.

⁑ *Try It: Chair Child's Pose with a Bolster*

Practice a variation of Child's Pose (Balasana) sitting in a chair.

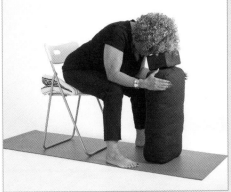

- In Child's Pose, there is benefit to making a connection between your forehead and the floor, but the connection may be lost if you need to practice in a chair. You can recreate that connection using props.
- Sit in a chair with your legs wide apart and place a bolster, standing on the short end, between your knees.
- Holding the bolster firmly with your hands, inhale and lengthen your spine, then hinge forward at your hips and try to rest your forehead on the top of the bolster. A block can be used to add height to the bolster.
- Notice the sensations of resting your forehead on the bolster or block.

Props Allow You to Release Effort

Props can support holding a pose for a longer period of time without muscular strength. This is one of the foundations of restorative yoga, where props are used to allow the body to rest in a pose rather than hold it in an engaged way. An example of this is supported Bridge Pose (Setu Bandha Sarvangasana), where you put a block or bolster under your sacrum. Bridge Pose can be challenging to hold for any length of time, but the support of the prop can help you hold it longer. Another great example of props allowing us to release effort is the use of a wall to support standing poses.

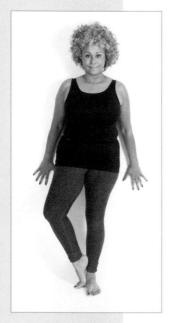

⠿ Try It: Tree Pose with a Wall ·······························

If you're able to stand, practice Tree Pose (Vrksasana) with your back against a wall to support you.

- Begin by standing with your back to the wall and a few inches away from it in Mountain Pose (Tadasana). Lean back and allow the wall to hold you as you shift your weight to your left leg with the knee slightly bent and the muscles engaged.
- Bend your right knee, and rotating at the hip, place the toes of your right foot on the floor alongside your left foot with your right heel against your left ankle.
- Bring your arms out to the side just slightly, and place your palms flat on the wall behind you. Notice how much easier it is to balance with your hands on the wall and how it allows you to release effort and relax into the pose.

·· ⠿

Props Can Apply Pressure

As I mentioned earlier, the floor is the most used and most underappreciated prop in asana practice. One important role of this "prop" is to massage the internal organs, in particular the digestive organs, by applying pressure during practice. However, if you're practicing in a chair, then the hard surface of the floor is only available for your feet. If you're practicing in bed, then the floor is replaced by the soft surface of the mattress, which can offer its own challenges. So in a chair or in bed, it may be necessary to recreate the pressure of the floor with other props.

You can try practicing a seated Cobra Pose with an emphasis on abdominal massage.

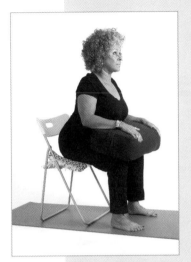

- Sitting in chair Mountain Pose (see page 25), place a bolster or folded blanket on your lap and rest your forearms over it, gently hugging it toward your abdomen.
- Bend forward from your hips and lower your head slightly.
- Exhale, and on your inhalation, slowly raise up into the pose by curling up your head, neck, and chest.
- Notice whether you feel a slight pressure from the bolster against your abdomen, giving you a gentle abdominal massage.
- Come out and notice how you feel.

DISSECT THE POSE

As you explore a new pose, it may be helpful to consider different aspects of what can be a complex experience. For example, in Tree Pose, which is a pose that may seem straightforward on the surface, many dynamics are actually happening at once. There's the experience of strengthening the supporting leg; hip opening in the bent leg; strengthening the core into a tall standing position; creating length in the spine; strengthening the raised, engaged arms; stretching in the shoulders; focusing the gaze; and concentrating the mind to allow for balance.

Additionally, the experience of grounding into the earth is essential for all standing poses—the way the breath allows the body to ground down on the exhalation and rebound upward on the inhalation. This is an important concept in asana practice, sending energy down into the earth in order for it to rise up.

It can be overwhelming to try to experience all of this at once, and it may not be physically comfortable or possible to create the traditional Tree Pose shape in your body. Instead, consider dissecting the pose into parts and practicing only one part at a time. To begin, can you focus on the grounded, strong, supporting leg?

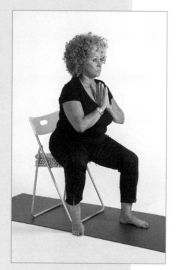

- Come to a tall chair Mountain Pose with your feet under your knees and your thighs parallel to the floor.
- Lean forward slightly and shift the weight of your body into your left leg, pressing your left foot into the floor to create a grounded feeling.
- Open your right leg out to your right side and lift your heel to balance on the ball of your right foot. Put your palms together at your chest.
- See if you can experience the grounding quality of Tree Pose in this seated position. Exhale, imagining the breath moving down your left leg onto the floor. Inhale, feeling the breath rebounding all the way up through your body.
- Release and notice how you feel.

· **::**

Change the Orientation

Some poses are challenging because of their orientation in space. For example, Downward-Facing Dog Pose (Adho Mukha Svanasana) can be a challenging practice for many people for multiple reasons, including not being able to have weight on their wrists. Instead you could practice a wall version of this pose where you bring your hands to the wall instead of the floor. Can you think of other poses where changing the orientation might make the practice more accessible?

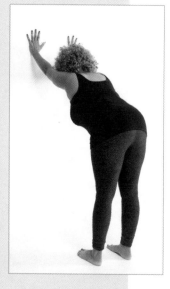

:: Try It: Practice Downward-Facing Dog Pose
   at the Wall ·

- Stand in Mountain Pose facing a wall and a little more than an arm's length away.
- Keeping your spine long, hinge at your hips and bring your hands to the wall at shoulder height.
- Keeping your head in line with the rest of your spine, move your tailbone away from the wall, finding length in your spine.
- You may need to play with the distance between your feet and the wall to find the ideal dimension.
- It's important not to sink into your shoulders but to keep your arms engaged.

- Similarly, it's important to keep your knees soft or slightly bent so that you don't hyperextend them.
- Hold for as long as you are comfortable and then slowly raise your head to come back to Mountain Pose.

Dynamic Practice

Another way to adapt asana is to practice in a dynamic way, coordinating the breath with the movement. Instead of holding a pose for a period of time (statically), there is constant movement. This is a great way to explore new poses in a safe way. It also can help quiet your mind by allowing you to explore the integration of breath and movement.

✛ Try It: Dynamic Cobra Pose

- *From a mat:* Lie on your abdomen with your legs stretched out and hip-width apart.
- Bring your forehead to the floor and place your hands under your shoulders with bent elbows.
- Inhale as you lift your head and chest, keeping your neck long and minimal weight on your hands.
- Then exhale as you slowly lower back down.
- Repeat a few times, seeing if you can connect your movement to your breath.

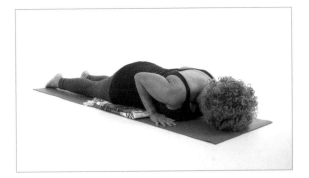
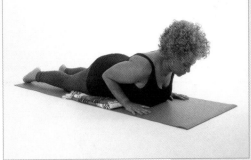

Imagine the Practice

Practicing asana just in the mind sounds like a really easy thing to do, and it does offer a way to practice for people who have limited mobility. Your body doesn't even have to move. But, interestingly, it is actually one of the most advanced forms of yoga practice, because it is only possible with a very concentrated mind. Recent studies of athletes have shown the benefits of visualizing their practice to improve performance and reduce anxiety.[10] This demonstrates how powerfully the body responds to what's happening in the mind. It also shows that practicing mentally is an excellent alternative to physical practice if you can keep your mind focused long enough to do it.

⁑ *Try It: Practice with Your Mind* ·

Think of your favorite yoga pose. If you can't think of any, try turning to a page in this book that has a photograph of a yoga pose.

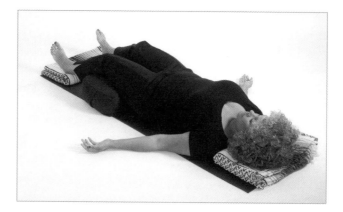

- Close your eyes. Imagine yourself preparing for the pose.
- Then as you inhale, imagine slowly coming into the pose.
- Hold the pose for a few breaths, imagining what you might be feeling in your body when doing the pose. Notice places where there is tension and places where there is opening.
- On an exhalation, slowly picture yourself coming out of the pose and relaxing.
- Notice how you feel after imagining the practice. Could you feel some benefit? Could you keep your mind focused long enough to engage in the practice?

· ⁑

Use Your Creativity

Asana practice is more about creativity than you might think. If you learn some of the essential elements of a particular asana, you can use your creativity to explore ways of practicing that feel safe and effective for your body. Of course, the creative aspect of yoga may come with self-confidence after a longer period of practice and study. But it's important not to lose the feeling of exploration and spontaneity; otherwise, your practice may become boring and stale.

✖ *Try It: Creative Cat/Cow Pose* ·

Try practicing Cat/Cow Pose (Marjaryasana/Bitilasana) with a focus on creative movement.

- This pose actually requires complex movements, as you move in and out of forward bending (spinal flexion) and backward bending (spinal extension) in a rhythmic, dynamic fashion.
- Practice either while sitting in a chair with your hands on your knees or on a mat on all fours, with your hands under your shoulders and your knees under your hips. Or, to avoid pressure on your wrists, you can place your forearms on a bolster.

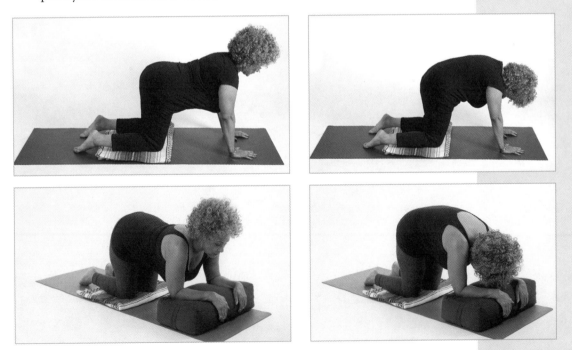

- In either position, begin by exhaling into a cat stretch, gently rounding your back and lowering your head.
- Then inhale into a cow stretch by arching your back and lifting your head.
- Now allow your body to move any way that feels comfortable, exploring the possible movements you can access from this position.
- See if you can engage your head, hips, and breath in a creative, spontaneous series of movements. You can even close your eyes if that's comfortable and allow yourself to move in any way that feels good in your body. This can be a useful way to explore the creative side of asana.
- Rest, and notice how you feel.

PART TWO

MAKING ASANA ACCESSIBLE

WARMING UP 3

AS YOU BEGIN to explore an Accessible Yoga practice, keep in mind that it may not look like the yoga you see on the covers of magazines. See if you can let go of preconceived ideas of what yoga is supposed to look like or feel like. Instead, focus on what you are actually experiencing in the moment. Begin by moving and exploring, reconnecting to your body—even the parts you don't like. Rather than judging yourself as "bad at yoga," see if you can simply observe how you feel. Notice how your body likes to move. See which practices feel good, and do more of those. Slowly build your practice.

CENTERING

Once you decide to practice yoga, your first question is, "How do I start?" Practice usually begins with some form of centering. This is the shifting of attention from the outer world to the inner world. Centering is about dropping into the space of neutral awareness, without judgment. In a way, centering is a microcosm for all of yoga. It's a process of quieting the noise in the mind so you can experience the truth beyond all the chaos.

Centering can take many forms, such as an extended Sanskrit chant in a more traditional yoga setting or a moment of silence and reflection. Here are a variety of techniques you could choose from when starting your practice. Explore different ones to find something that feels comfortable and effective for you so that you can create a conscious way to begin your practice.

OUTER SENSING

Sensing is a process of consciously connecting to the input you're receiving through your senses. Can you pause for a moment and notice the pressure of your feet against the floor, the texture of your clothing, or the temperature of the air on your skin? What sounds do you hear? What do you see? What do you smell? Do you feel safe and comfortable?

INNER SENSING

Focus on interoception. What is happening in your body? Are there sensations in your bones, joints, muscles, organs? Is there energy in your body? Do you feel tired or awake, hungry or full, hot or cold? Are there emotions in your body? Also notice if you can sense where your body is in space (proprioceptive awareness). What position are your legs and arms in? This is not a time to judge your posture or your body in general; rather, it's a time to notice an internal world of sensation and experience.

For some people, especially those in chronic pain, this can be a painful experience. Be sure to use your judgment, and don't push yourself beyond your limits. If increased internal awareness is painful, choose a different technique.

POSTURE CHECK

As part of the centering process, take a moment to check your posture and see if you can lengthen your spine. To do this, you can exhale and feel energy moving down into the earth. On the next inhalation, feel energy rising up from the earth through your body, lengthening your spine all the way up through your neck to the top of your head.

Sitting in a Chair

Choose a sturdy chair for your practice that has a firm seat and, if possible, no arms. Posture check in a chair is also called chair Mountain Pose, which can be done with your arms out to the sides or with your hands together in prayer position (*namaste*). You can take your shoes off or leave them on if that's more comfortable for you, although practicing barefoot is beneficial to your nervous system. Start by noticing if your feet easily reach the floor. If not, try placing a folded blanket under your feet so your knees are just slightly lower than, or level with, your hips. If your knees are higher than your hips, consider placing a folded blanket on the seat of the chair under your sit bones to elevate your hips.

If you need to lean against the back of the chair, try to sit as far back on the seat as possible so that the back supports an elongated spine and tall posture. If you need extra support to keep your body upright and there's a danger of falling out of the chair, consider placing a strap around the back of the chair and all the way around your waist like a seatbelt. Or bring your feet slightly forward of your knees, which can prevent you from falling forward.

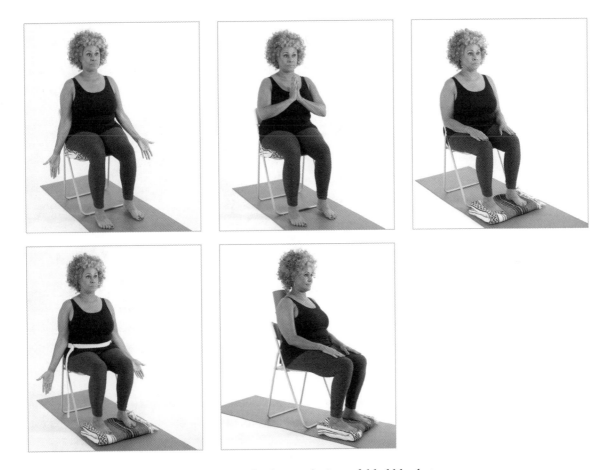

To support kyphosis, a rounded upper back, try placing a folded blanket or small pillow behind your upper back and lean into it. Or you can use a rolled yoga mat behind your back. Roll the mat loosely if you want to make it a little softer, and place it directly behind and parallel to your spine, from the midback up to the back of your head.

The goal of these props is to help you lengthen your spine and create a posture where your chest is expanded, your shoulders are back and down, and your neck is long. As part of the posture check, you can close your eyes or simply relax them, and notice how your body feels. Be aware of your breath as well as any thoughts and emotions in the mind.

Sitting on the Floor

If you're sitting on the floor, you can explore using props to make yourself more comfortable. You can sit on a cushion, bolster, block, or pillow. By elevating your seat in this way, you create more space in your hips and allow

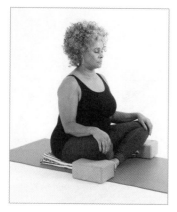
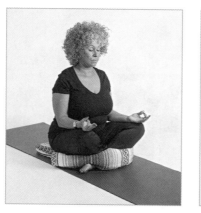
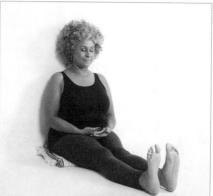

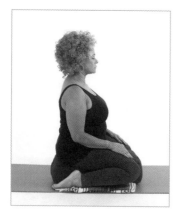

for a gentle curve in your lower back. Supporting your knees can be very helpful in relieving some pressure on your hips in a cross-legged position.

You can either place blocks under your knees or, taking a blanket and rolling it into a long log shape, place it between your feet and knees. This can relieve the pressure on your feet and simultaneously lift your knees. If your back is uncomfortable, try sitting on a higher support or extending your legs out in front of you. You can sit with your back against a wall for extra support.

Remember the goal is to sit comfortably and have a long spine. If sitting cross-legged is uncomfortable, you can sit in a variation of Thunderbolt Pose (Vajrasana). Kneel on a blanket with your toes coming off the back. Place a bolster, cushion, or block under your sit bones. The support can be between your knees or behind your thighs, whichever is more comfortable for you.

Lying in Bed

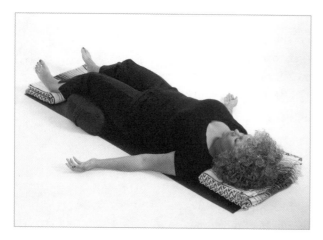

If you're practicing yoga in bed, you can check your posture in Corpse Pose (Savasana). Lie with your legs outstretched and your arms out to the sides. Place a small pillow or folded blanket under your head. If possible, have your forehead level with, or slightly higher than, your chin.

Avoid using a firm pillow that lifts your head high. Instead, focus on supporting a gentle curve in the back of your neck. If there's discomfort in your lower back when your legs are straight, then you can place a bolster, rolled blanket, or folded pillow under your knees.

Standing

Most of the warm-ups in this section can be practiced from a standing position if that's more comfortable for you. In yoga, the basic standing pose is called Mountain Pose, which is the foundation for all the other standing poses.

In Mountain Pose, one of the most important elements is grounding down into the earth. This is done by connecting with the feeling of your feet on the floor and the feeling of energy moving down as you exhale. This downward-moving energy then rebounds up through your body to lift and lengthen your spine as you inhale.

You can practice Mountain Pose with your back against a wall or holding on to the back of a chair for extra support. Have your knees soft and your thighs engaged. Your shoulders are back and relaxed; your head is centered with your chin parallel to the floor.

INTENTION

Take a moment to set an intention for your practice. What are you trying to find: peace of mind, a release of anxiety, stress reduction, improved health, or connection with your body? Whatever your intention, it can be useful to spend a moment before you begin practice to bring this into your mind.

If there is something you're working on in your life, something you're confused about, or a decision you have to make, it can be useful to ask

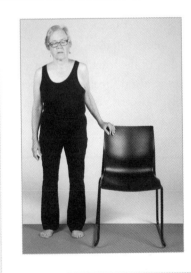

Judy Hubbell:
Standing Mountain Pose Holding Chair

"For standing Mountain Pose, I close my eyes, lengthen through the three areas of my spine, feel the grounding of my feet, imagine energy traveling up and down through my body, and bring my chin level to the floor, sometimes with a chair as an assist. Although one hip is higher than the other and one leg longer, I am then very comfortable doing a full Sun Salutation, remembering this lengthening process on the forward bend as I move away from the chair and return to the mat."

yourself a question before you begin to practice. Then let it go and see what comes up as you connect with your body and breath—as you begin to move and breathe. Through practice, we can begin to access our intuition or inner wisdom.

Breath Meditation

Meditating on your breath can be a very effective centering technique since the breath is an ever-present object for concentration. Observing the movement of the breath, or experiencing the sensation of breathing, is very effective for quieting the mind. I'll discuss breathing practices and meditation in more detail later in the book. If you've had trauma, anxiety, or depression, it can be helpful to keep your eyes open during meditation and gaze at something neutral like a candle flame or flower, or relax the focus of your eyes instead of closing them.

Body Scan

Another option is to do a body scan, or guided relaxation, noticing sensations in each part of your body in a directed, conscious way. Move your awareness from your feet to your head or your head to your feet. By connecting with sensations in your body, you can shift your awareness away from the busy mind back into the present moment. I'll talk more about the techniques of guided relaxation, Corpse Pose, and yoga nidra later in the book.

Centering through Sound

The traditional centering practice of yoga is Sanskrit chanting. These chants, which are usually an invocation of the guru or of the teachings themselves, can give you the opportunity to transcend the mind through the power of sound vibration. If you're not familiar with Sanskrit chants, an effective option is to use other forms of sound vibration. Here are some different ways to use sound vibration as a centering practice.

Singing

Try singing a folk song like "Row, Row, Row Your Boat," or any song that is uplifting and fun, to experience the benefits of sound vibration. Singing is also a form of pranayama, expanding and deepening the breath.

Vocalizing

Making other kinds of vocalizations can also be effective. For example, taking a deep inhalation, and then saying a long slow "Ah" on the exhalation can be very effective in using the power of sound, quieting the mind, and turning awareness inward.

Dissected OM

These days it's normal to hear OM chanted in every yoga class. OM is a Sanskrit word that represents all the sound vibration in the entire universe. You can chant three OMs out loud or silently in your mind. When chanting OM, try to focus on the "mm" part of the sound and have your teeth gently touching so you can feel the vibration in your head. You could also try separating out the three syllables of the word into

"Aaaahhhh"
"Ooooooo"
"Mmmmm"

Bowls or Bells

Crystal singing bowls, bells, or other types of instruments are effective at quieting the mind by offering an external sound to focus on.

Music

Calm music can be very effective for relaxing the mind. But it's useful to spend some silent time in your practice as well.

MUDRAS

Mudras are gestures that are used for a variety of purposes in the yoga tradition. They can stimulate certain pressure points in the body, or they can allow energy (prana) to recirculate in the body. They can also represent aspects of nature or deities in the Hindu tradition. Mudras can be a useful centering practice, especially if you're deaf or hard of hearing and chanting isn't effective for you.

when working in that area. Generally, severe inflammation needs to heal before movement is reintroduced.

EYE MOVEMENTS

Working with the eyes is a good way to learn how to connect movement with breath and consciously turn the awareness from the outer world to the inner world. You can explore the physical structure of the eye in this practice rather than focus on the sensory stimulation that seeing people receive through the eyes. The eyes are also closely connected to the brain, and stored memories can be released through these types of movements. For these reasons, eye movements need to be approached with care.

Vertical and Horizontal

Coordinate the movements of your eyes with your breath. For example, inhale and look up, exhale and look down. Or inhale and look left, exhale and look right. Repeat vertical movements a few times, pause, and then do a few horizontal movements.

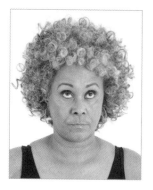
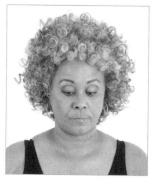

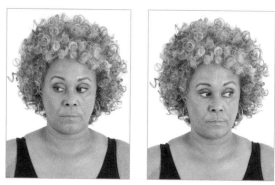

Trace a Circle

Following your hand with your eyes, slowly draw a circle in front of you. The circle can be just at the edge of your vision. Inhale as your eyes go up, exhale as they go down. After a few circles, close your eyes. Then repeat in the opposite direction.

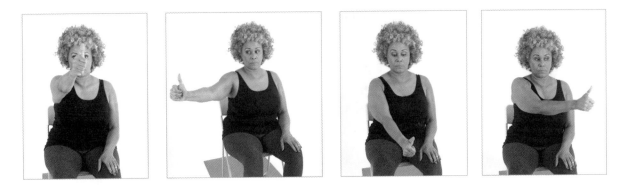

Trace a Square

Looking across the room, trace a square by following the lines of the wall in front of you. Look across the ceiling, down at the corner of the wall, across the floor, and up the other corner. Or trace a window with your eyes. Start going in one direction. Pause and close your eyes. Then go in the opposite direction.

Palming

After any of these eye movements, or by itself, palming is a soothing practice for the eyes. Rub your hands together briskly to create heat. If you have the use of only one hand, you can rub it on your thigh. Then place your warmed palms (or palm) over your eyes. When the heat dissipates, you can gently massage your eyes. Repeat once more.

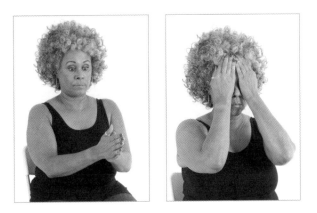

SHOULDER CIRCLES

From a chair, mat, or standing: Coordinating the breath and movement, inhale as your shoulders come up toward your ears and slowly roll back, as if they could meet behind you. Then as you exhale, continue to roll your shoulders down and then forward, creating a full circle. This movement engages the chest, upper back, and neck muscles rather than the shoulder joint itself. After a few circles, reverse directions.

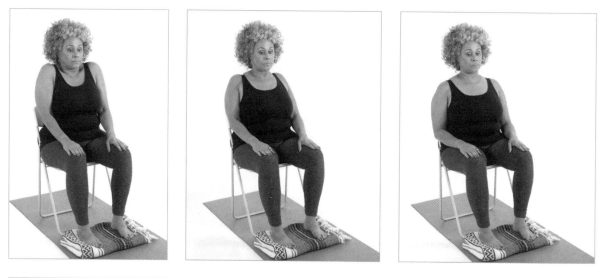

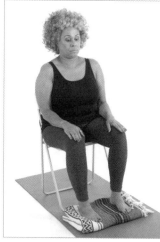

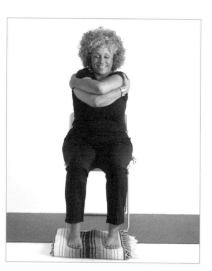

HUG

From a chair, bed, mat, or standing: Give yourself a hug, taking hold of opposite shoulders. Spend a moment giving yourself some love. Then switch your arms so the other one is on top.

ARM RAISES

From a chair: Bring your arms out to the sides of your body with your palms facing up. Imagine your breath is like helium, and imagine you're filling your arms with helium as you inhale. Observe your arms lifting, as if on their own, just from the power of your breath. Once you reach the top of your range of motion, exhale, turn your palms down, and allow your arms to float down slowly. Repeat a few times, continuing to focus on your breath.

From a bed or mat: A similar practice can be done by stretching your arms out in a T shape. Then inhale and lift your arms toward the ceiling, bringing your palms together overhead. Turn your palms away from each other, and as you exhale, slowly lower them back to the floor or bed.

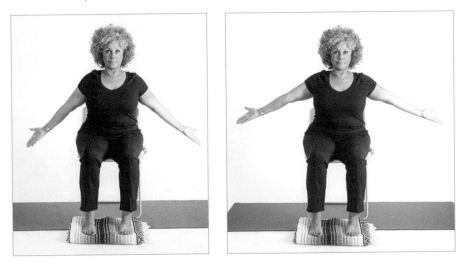

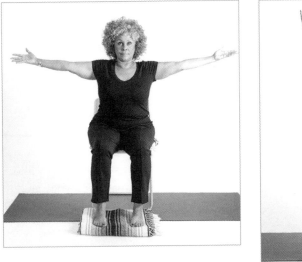

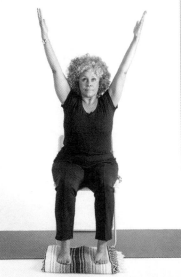

PICKING CHERRIES

From a chair: Imagine you're picking cherries off a high tree branch. Start in chair Mountain Pose. Reach up with one arm, imagining you're picking cherries and putting them in a basket on the other side of your body. Coordinate with your breath, inhaling as your arm goes up and exhaling as it comes down. Practice a few times and then switch sides.

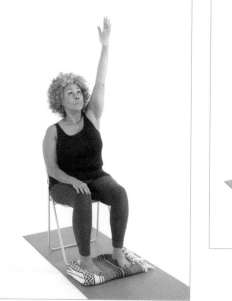

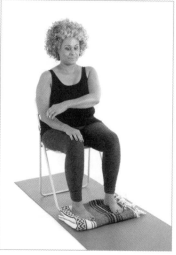

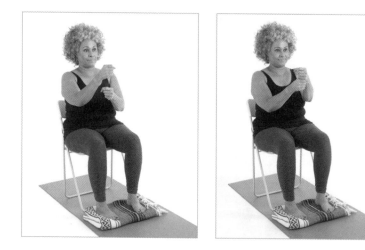

CLIMBING ROPE

From a chair, bed, or mat: Pretend you're climbing a rope in front of you by reaching out with one hand at a time and holding an imaginary rope. Engage your hands, arms, and chest without straining, and find a way to coordinate with your breath. See how high you can climb without straining.

WRIST/HAND MOVEMENTS

From a chair or mat: With your arms out in front of you at shoulder height, try moving your hands into different positions and make correlated animal noises, as described here.

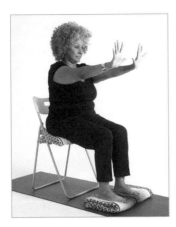

Webs

Raise your hands, flex your wrists, and stretch your fingers wide apart as if making webbed feet. Make a frog sound as you do so.

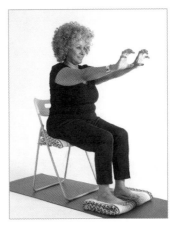

Claws

With your hands up, curl your fingers and thumbs into claws as you make a roaring sound like a tiger.

Beaks

Bring your fingers together and, keeping them straight, move them toward and away from your thumbs like duck bills as you make a duck sound.

Paws

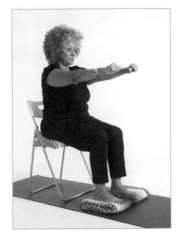

Make gentle fists with your thumbs on the outside, as if they are puppy paws. Bend your wrists up and down as you make a panting dog sound.

If your arms get tired, you can practice these exercises with your elbows bent and your arms close to your body. These movements can also be practiced lying down with your arms stretched toward the ceiling or with your elbows bent and your upper arms resting on the floor alongside your body.

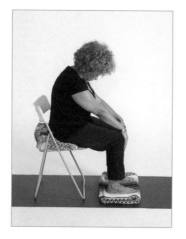

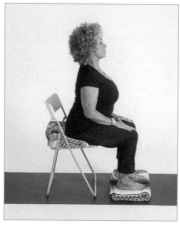

Cat/Cow Pose

From a chair: Avoid doing this type of spinal flexion (rounding of the back) if you have osteoporosis. Exhale and round your back like a cat, as you slide your hands down your knees, making claws with your fingers. Inhale, lift your chest, and allow the middle of your back to move forward into a cow shape. If you like, you can add a "meow" sound on the cat movement and a "moo" on the cow movement. Continue, following your breath for a few rounds.

Cat/Cow Pose on All Fours

From a mat: Come to your hands and knees. You can place a blanket under your knees to protect them. Exhale, lift your midback toward the ceiling, and lower your head. Inhale, raise your head, and allow your abdomen and chest to move toward the floor. Let the movement flow through your spine in a rhythmic movement that follows your breath.

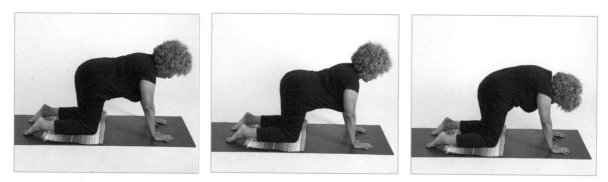

Cat/Cow Pose with Bolster

From a mat: If your wrists are uncomfortable on the floor, you can place one or two bolsters under your forearms to avoid straining your wrists in this pose. Or you can use the seat of a chair in front of you in a similar way. Exhale and round your back like a cat, lifting your midback toward the ceiling and lowering your head. Inhale, lower your chest and belly, let your chest move forward, and raise your head into a cow shape. Continue, following your breath for a few rounds.

Cat/Cow Pose can also be turned into a creative exploration of movement. Consider moving your spine sideways or making hip circles. Use your creativity to find actions that bring movement into the core of your body—the spine, pelvis, hips, and shoulders.

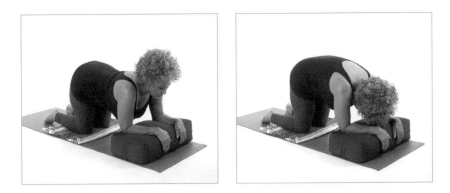

Foot Movements

From a chair, bed, or mat: Extend your feet out in front of you. If you're sitting in a chair, you can rest your feet on the floor or a bolster on the floor in front of you. Slowly point and flex your feet, being careful to avoid cramping. You can try to spread your toes apart and then squeeze them together. Explore other foot movements such as circling your feet or pretending to draw letters in the air with your toes. You can also roll your feet from side to side like windshield wipers. Try to coordinate all these movements with your breath.

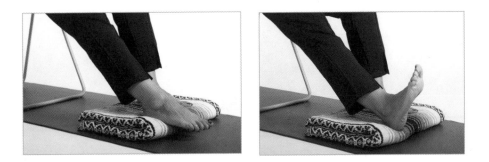

STRENGTHENING AND MASSAGING 4

PRACTICING YOGA in a chair or in bed can offer many of the same benefits as practicing in a traditional way on the floor. These benefits include physically stretching muscles, tendons, and fascia, as well as learning to stimulate the relaxation response in the nervous system. But there are a few benefits that may be lost when asana is adapted in this way, unless you specifically target them in your chair or bed practice.

One important benefit that may be lost is the strengthening quality of many yoga poses. In particular, the weight-bearing aspect of poses like Downward-Facing Dog Pose or standing balancing poses. Weight-bearing poses are particularly useful for people with osteoporosis, which causes severely weakened bone structure, as well as its precursor, osteopenia, and those at risk for osteoporosis. We tend to think of bones as the inert skeleton that supports the dynamic muscles and organs. But bones are vital, living structures, and like muscles they respond to challenges by getting stronger.

Another benefit that may be lost in a chair or bed practice is the deep massage to the digestive organs and other systems of the body. Yoga teachers have long made various, and sometimes suspicious, claims about the health benefits of yoga. But it doesn't take much of a scientific background to feel how pressure on the belly can help stimulate the digestive organs.

Many poses put pressure on the abdomen, either against the floor or against the arms or legs. Twisting poses can also offer this digestive massage. But many people will benefit from adding specific self-massage techniques in a chair or bed practice. Here are some ideas for incorporating strengthening and massaging practices into your routine.

STRENGTHENING: UPPER BODY

To strengthen your upper body, you may first want to consider that there are a few different ways to strengthen muscles, including isometric exercise, where the muscle doesn't change length (such as holding Plank Pose

[Kumbhakasana]), and isotonic exercise, where the muscles get longer and shorter (moving dynamically in and out of a pose). You can do both with yoga, which we will explore here.

Here are some benefits of strengthening practices:

- Increase overall strength
- Increase bone density
- Increase stability

When practicing in a chair or in bed, you can find a variety of ways to strengthen your upper body—arms, shoulders, chest, back, and core muscles. It's important to keep the breath steady when working with these practices. Holding your breath can be a sign that you're straining. Here are just a few examples of strengthening practices that may be particularly helpful with creating stability in the body. I hope you'll explore different ways to strengthen your body from seated or prone positions.

It's important to approach these strengthening practices with energy and enthusiasm, because muscles and bones get stronger when they are challenged. The issue is that you don't want to strain and cause an injury or experience extreme soreness the next day. So the question becomes: How can you challenge yourself to get stronger without causing injury? If you are not currently exercising, it's important to go very slowly. Rather than holding a position in a static way, try coming in and out of it with the breath. Once you're more confident, you can hold it longer, up to ten or more breath cycles. If these practices feel too easy, you might want to try incorporating light handheld weights in your practice so you can continue to get stronger.

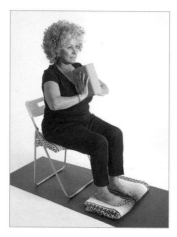

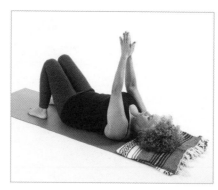

Chest Press

From a chair or bed: Explore isometric strengthening practices by pressing your hands together in front of your chest or pressing your hands into a block held at chest level.

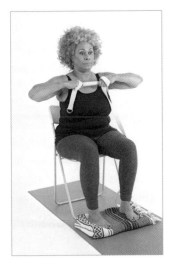

Chest Pull

From a chair or bed: Hold a strap gently in both hands and pull your hands away from each other. Engage the muscles in your arms, shoulders, and chest.

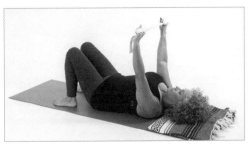

Arm Hold

From a chair: Hold your arms out at shoulder height, either out to the sides or in front of your body.

　From a bed: Extend your arms out to the sides and lift them just above the surface of the bed. Keep your breath steady.

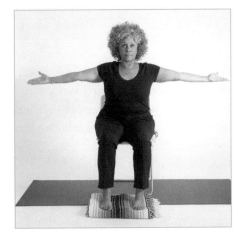

Chair Lift and Press

From a chair: Holding the sides of the chair seat, pull up, engaging the muscles in your arms and shoulders. Keep your spine long and focus on the muscles that are working. Then press your hands into the seat, feeling your spine lengthen and your head lift. Keep your breath relaxed. This movement can be coordinated with your breath.

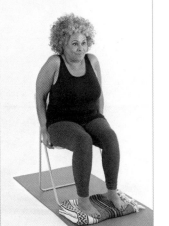
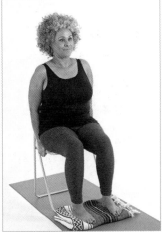

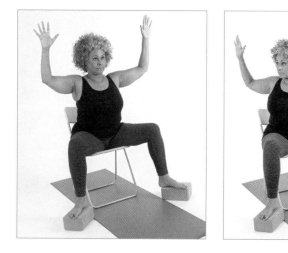

Goddess Twist

From a chair: From chair Mountain Pose, widen your legs and place your feet flat on the floor, or on blocks to increase the stretch in your inner thighs and hips. Raise your arms out to the sides and bend your elbows. Inhale and lengthen your spine. Exhale as you twist to the right. Inhale as you come back to neutral. Exhale and twist to the left. Continue for a few rounds.

STRENGTHENING: LOWER BODY

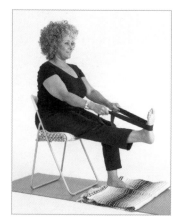

Leg Lifts

From a chair: Hold your right thigh, or hold a strap that's around your right foot. Extend your right leg out in front of you, straightening the leg. If this is comfortable, hold for a few breaths. While holding, you can flex and point your foot. Try coordinating your foot movements with your breath.

From a bed or mat: Bend both knees and place your feet flat on the mat or bed. Then slowly lift your left leg, bending the knee, inhale, and bring your leg toward your chest. As you exhale, straighten your leg and slowly lower it down toward the floor. Be careful not to strain your back. Use your arms to help if needed. Repeat with the other leg.

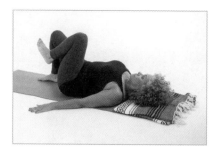

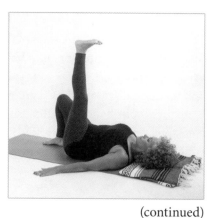

(continued)

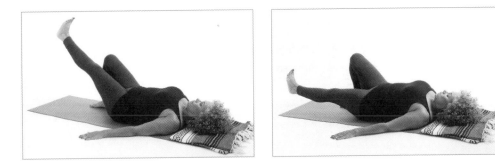

Knee Press

From a chair or bed: With your knees bent, place a block between your knees. Press into the block equally with both legs. Keep your breath relaxed.

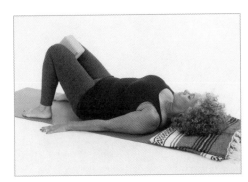

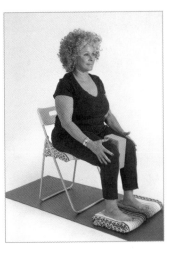

Knees Apart

From a chair or bed: Place a strap gently around both thighs. Try opening your knees, pressing your thighs into the strap. Or, bring your hands to the outside of your thighs and open your legs, resisting with your hands.

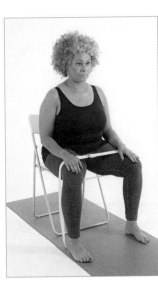

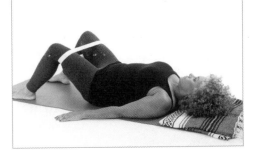

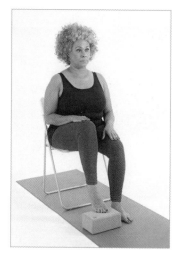

Calf Strengthener

From a chair or bed: With your knees bent, place the toes of one foot on a block. Lift the heel and then lower it. Coordinate with your breath, but be careful not to cause a cramp in your foot. This can also be done by placing your heel on a block and pointing and flexing your foot in order to increase the range of motion in your foot. Repeat with the other foot.

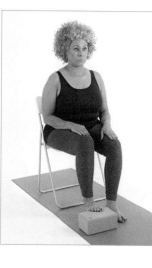

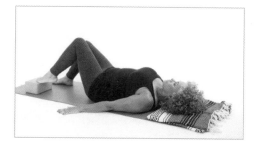

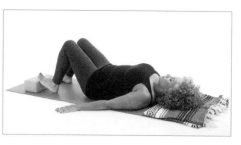

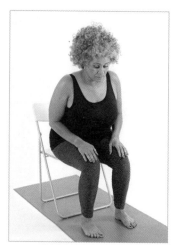

Sit to Stand

From a chair: Hold the sides of the chair seat or have your hands on your knees.. Lean forward, press your feet into the floor, and engage all the muscles in your legs as you shift your weight forward. The movement is the same as if you're about to stand up. If you have the strength in your legs, you can lift your buttocks slightly off the chair seat and then sit back down.

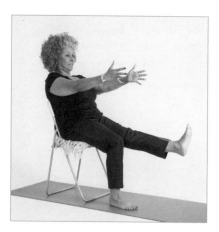

Boat Pose (Navasana)

From a chair: This pose helps to strengthen the abdominal and core muscles. Make sure that you're secure in the chair and not straining in this pose. To begin, lean back in the chair and extend one leg, holding the seat of the chair or the back of your thigh. Once you're feeling steady and comfortable, you can stretch your arms out in front of you. Take a few breaths and then switch sides.

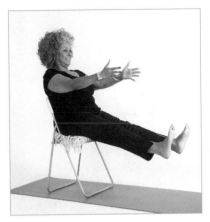

From a chair: If this is very comfortable, you can try to lift both legs at the same time, but be sure not to strain and try not to hold your breath. *Contraindication:* Do not lift both feet off the floor if there is a fall risk.

From a mat: Sit on the floor with your legs extended in front of you. Place a bolster under your calves. Begin to lean back, hinging at your hips and keeping your spine long and your breath relaxed. Rest your lower legs on the bolster and hold for a few breaths, or as long as comfortable without straining. This pose can also be done with your feet on the wall.

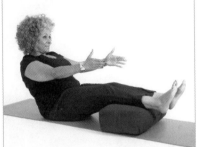

SELF-MASSAGE

Self-massage is an important self-care practice that can help release tension and increase blood flow and lymph circulation. You can massage your body gently using your own hands, unless this is painful because of arthritis or carpal tunnel syndrome. If using your hands is painful, you can use a tennis ball or foam roller for self-massage.

Neck Squeeze

From a chair or bed: Interlace your fingers behind your head. Use your thumbs to gently massage the base of your skull.

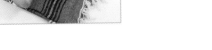

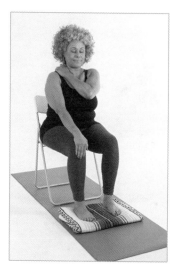

Shoulder Rub

From a chair or bed: Massage one shoulder with the opposite hand. Repeat on the opposite side.

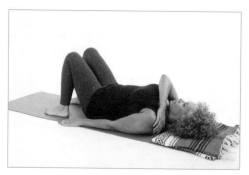

Lymphatic Massage

From a chair, bed, or mat: Gently stroke your arms and legs toward your trunk, in the direction of the heart, to stimulate lymphatic drainage. Lymph is the fluid of the immune system, and it relies on diaphragmatic breathing and movement to flow through the body.

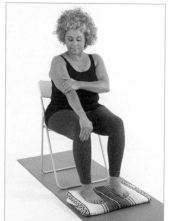

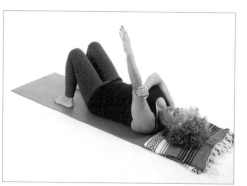

Abdominal Massage

From a chair, bed, or mat: Massage your abdomen up on the right side, across the middle, and down on the left. If you're looking down at your abdomen, this is a clockwise motion. You can use the heel of your hand, with your other hand on top for added pressure. Keep your breath relaxed, and begin gently. If it's comfortable, you can press a little harder. Abdominal massage is an essential part of asana practice because of the importance of digestive health. In particular, it can help with bloating or constipation by stimulating peristalsis in the large intestine.

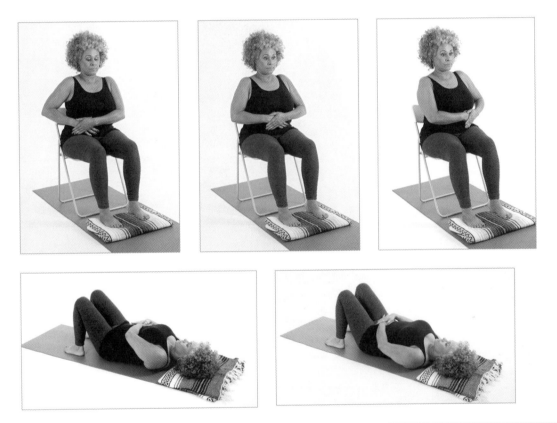

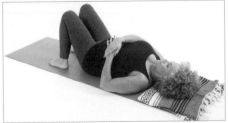

SUN SALUTATION 5

SUN SALUTATION is an effective way to warm up your entire body, whether as preparation for more poses or simply to warm yourself up on a cold morning. It's also a powerful practice on its own that can help you connect with your breath and the rhythmic movements of nature.

Sun Salutation can be made more accessible in a number of ways. You can either practice a variation of a traditional Sun Salutation series by adapting the individual positions within it, or you can remove poses or sections of the series that present the greatest challenge. Other ways to adapt the sequence include using props, such as a wall or chair, as well as practicing in bed or lying on a mat.

Here are the main benefits of practicing Sun Salutation:

- Warming up the entire body
- Linking breath and movement
- Creating a ritual, a series of movements that you can link together and repeat regularly
- Connecting to nature

WALL SUN SALUTATION

Practicing Sun Salutation at the wall is extremely helpful if you don't want to get down on the floor or you can't easily reach the floor with your hands. This can also be useful if you don't want to put weight on your knees, if you want to reduce the weight on your wrists or shoulders, or if you're in an airport and don't want to touch the floor! It's also useful for pregnant women because it eliminates pressure on the belly.

If you don't have wall space available, or if you want to avoid bending your wrists, the same wall Sun Salutation series that follows can be done using the back or the seat of a chair instead of a wall. But make sure that the chair is very stable, either by placing it against a wall, on top of a yoga mat, or both.

This series can be adapted to match whatever version of Sun Salutation you may already be practicing by using the wall in the same way you use the floor. For example, you could replace one of the wall Downward-Facing Dog poses with a wall Plank Pose. Use your creativity, and remember the key element is combining the movements with your breath.

To prepare, place your mat perpendicular to a wall, with one of the short edges of the mat touching the wall. Stand facing the wall, slightly farther than arm's length away, with your feet hip-width apart.

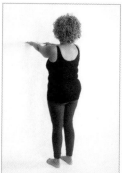
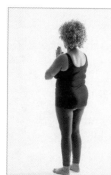

1. Inhale and bring your palms together in front of your chest. Then exhale.

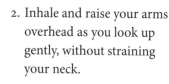

2. Inhale and raise your arms overhead as you look up gently, without straining your neck.

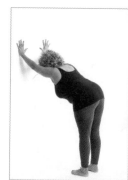

3. Exhale and hinge forward from your hips, placing your palms on the wall at shoulder height into wall Downward-Facing Dog Pose (see page 112).

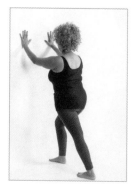

4. Inhale and step your right foot forward, bringing your toes up to the wall and bending your right knee. Keep your left leg straight. Press your chest away from the wall and lengthen your spine upward. Look up slightly.

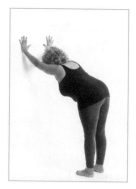

5. Exhale, step your right foot back to be parallel with your left foot, hip-width apart, into wall Downward-Facing Dog Pose.

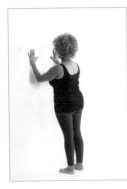

6. Inhale, raising your torso, and step both feet forward, halfway to the wall; bend your arms slightly. Exhale and engage your arms muscles.

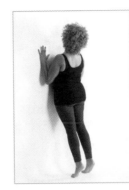

7. Inhale, bend your arms, and press your chest toward the wall as you come up onto your toes. Lift your chin, coming into a slight backbend. Keep your neck long without dropping your head back.

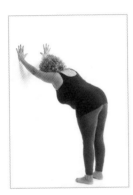

8. Exhale, lower your heels back to the floor, and step both feet back, hinging forward into wall Downward-Facing Dog Pose.

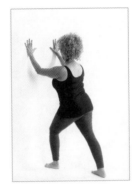

9. Inhale, step your left foot forward and bend your left knee, keeping your right leg straight. Press your chest away from the wall. Lengthen your spine, looking up gently.

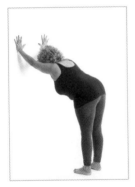

10. Exhale, step your left foot back to be parallel with your right foot, hip-width apart, into wall Downward-Facing Dog Pose.

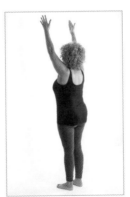

11. Inhale and raise your head. Push off from the wall, keeping your arms lifted overhead. Look up gently.

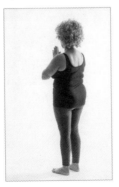

12. Exhale and lower your arms. Bring your palms together at your chest.

Chair Sun Salutation

Sun Salutation can also be done as a seated practice, which takes a little more imagination. There are two ways to approach the practice. One is to try to align movements in the chair with the traditional standing Sun Salutation so they could be practiced side by side. Another approach is to be more creative with the movements and focus on moving with the breath, getting as many major muscle groups involved as possible.

Generally, try to inhale when you bend back (spinal extension) and exhale when you bend forward (spinal or hip flexion). Sun Salutation is, by definition, a series of flowing movements coordinated with the breath. Use your imagination, and see what type of chair Sun Salutation you can create. The chair can be against a wall for support or on a yoga mat to provide more traction. When practicing in a chair, be careful to keep the bulk of your weight in the chair to avoid falling out of it.

For many people, chair Sun Salutation offers a way to continue a much-loved practice in the face of injury or illness. The flow of breath and movement is soothing to the mind and nervous system, and it can help bring us back to the body during times of anxiety or stress. I remember one student with multiple sclerosis who was dealing with extreme fatigue. Some days she had enough energy to practice a standing Sun Salutation, and some days she preferred to sit in a chair. But either way she was able to experience this powerful moving meditation.

To begin, come to chair Mountain Pose, feet firmly planted on the floor with your knees over your ankles and your thighs parallel to the floor. (For shorter legs, place a blanket or block under your feet. For longer legs, sit on a folded blanket). Sit toward the front of the chair with your spine long.

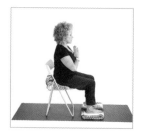 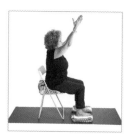 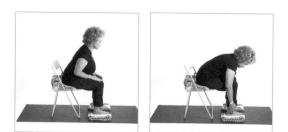

1. Exhale and bring your palms together in front of your chest.

2. Inhale, extend your arms out in front, and stretch them up over your head; look up gently.

3. Exhale, lower your hands to your thighs, and hinge forward at your hips, keeping your neck and spine long. Slide your hands down your legs toward your feet. Relax your neck.

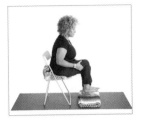 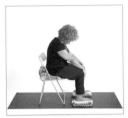 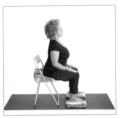 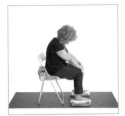

4. Inhale and slowly rise up. Take hold of your right thigh and lift it toward your abdomen in a modified lunge. Move your chest forward and look ahead.

5. Exhale and release your leg; return your hands to your knees. Round your back and lower your head into a seated Cat Pose.

6. Inhale, move your chest forward, and look up, coming into a seated Cow Pose.

7. Exhale and round your back into a seated Cat Pose.

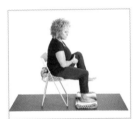 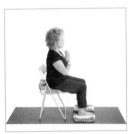

8. Inhale and rise up. Take hold of your left thigh and lift it toward your abdomen. Move your chest forward and look ahead.

9. Exhale and release your leg. Lower your hands to your thighs, and hinge forward at your hips, keeping your neck and spine long. Slide your hands down your legs toward your feet and relax your neck.

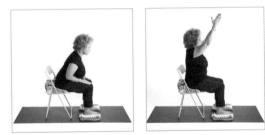 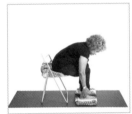

10. Inhale and place your hands back on your thighs. Lengthen your neck and come up with a long spine. Raise your arms up overhead and look up gently.

11. Exhale and bring your palms together in front of your chest.

Bed Sun Salutation

The energetic flow of Sun Salutation can be experienced lying in bed or lying on a mat. Use your creativity to explore what movements feel good in your body. Working from this position, gravity affects the body in a different way. Notice how raising your arms in front of you creates a similar experience as raising them over your head in a seated position.

The movements in this flow tend to focus on hip and shoulder opening, which can be a great practice if you're spending a lot of time in bed. This includes people with chronic illness, fatigue, before or after surgery, and so on.

Begin by checking your posture in bed; this is a variation of Corpse Pose focusing on comfort and stability. You can begin with both knees bent and your feet on the bed.

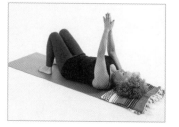

1. Exhale and bring your palms together at your chest.

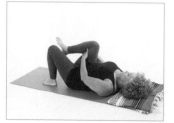
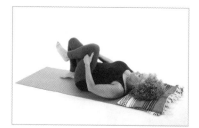

2. Inhale as you raise your arms toward the ceiling, then open your arms out to the sides.

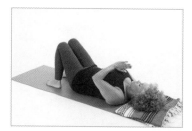

3. Exhale and raise your arms back toward the ceiling, then bring your hands back down to your chest.

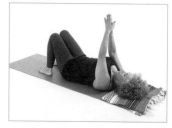

4. Inhale, take hold of your right leg behind the thigh, and bring your head toward your right knee. Exhale and release your head and leg.

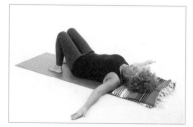

5. Inhale, take hold of your left leg behind the thigh, and raise your head toward your left knee. Exhale and release your head and leg.

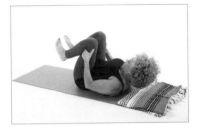

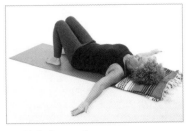

6. Inhale, hug both knees in toward your chest, and raise your head. Exhale and release your head and legs.

7. Inhale, and open your arms out to the sides.

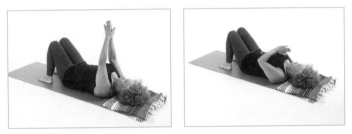

8. Exhale and raise your arms back toward the ceiling, then bring your hands back down to your chest.

With creativity, Sun Salutation can be practiced and explored at the wall, seated, or in bed—maybe even in other ways. You can practice it sitting on a mat with your legs out in front of you or kneeling. Within the practice, there is so much potential to explore flowing, rhythmic movements. You can even create your own rhythm by putting together a few poses that flow nicely.

STANDING AND BALANCING 6

STANDING POSES offer so many benefits, both physical and mental: they can improve posture and balance, as well as increase concentration and strength. There is a certain quality to standing poses that gives the feeling of being grounded and strong. Grounding is a hard quality to define, but it is the feeling of being firmly planted on the earth. In order to stand, on either one or two feet, we need to be firmly connected to the ground.

You can explore variations of standing poses in a chair, in bed, and lying or sitting on a mat. When practicing standing poses lying on a mat or in bed, consider ways to experience grounding. Often pressure on the soles of the feet and the palms of the hands can bring that feeling of connecting with the earth. Another way to feel grounded when lying down is to have weight on the body, such as a heavy blanket or a bolster on the chest.

The main benefits of standing balancing poses are:

- Strength
- Balance
- Grounding

STANDING MOUNTAIN POSE (TADASANA)

Mountain Pose is considered the foundation pose for all standing poses. If you're unsteady on your feet, then Mountain Pose becomes a challenging balancing pose, and tips for balancing poses can be applied. For example, using a *drishti*, or focus for the eyes, can greatly improve your balance in Mountain Pose. Try focusing on a point on the floor just a few feet away from you. Over time you can look farther out across the room, with the emphasis on fixing your eyes on one point. This is a great practice for concentrating the mind as well.

Begin practicing standing Mountain Pose by bringing your awareness to your feet, which can be about hip-width apart. If you're barefoot, try lifting

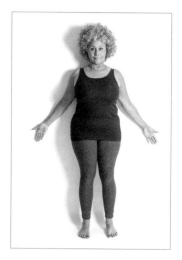

and spreading your toes, and then lift and lower your heels. Feel your weight shifting forward and back, and try to find center. Then shift your weight gently from right to left to find center again. Bend your knees slightly to engage your thigh muscles. Inhale, and lengthen your spine all the way up through the top of your head, allowing for the natural curves of the spine. Exhale and relax your shoulders back and down with your arms out at the sides and palms toward the hips or facing forward. Allow your face to be relaxed. Take a few breaths here, focusing on the feeling of your breath moving up and down your body, grounding and lifting at the same time.

Mountain Pose with Back to Wall

From standing: If you feel unsteady standing on both feet, you can use support. Begin by practicing Mountain Pose with your back against the wall. To cultivate the experience of grounding, try bringing your arms alongside your body and pressing your palms into the wall.

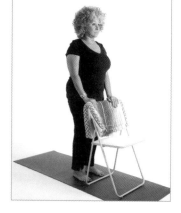

Mountain Pose Holding a Chair

From standing: Standing behind a chair and holding on to the back can offer needed support to avoid falling. In these variations, work on consciously connecting the soles of your feet to the ground (if possible, practice in bare feet). Some people find it easier to balance with their feet directly on the floor rather than on a yoga mat. See what feels most effective for you.

As you practice this pose, you can also work toward releasing your grip on the wall or the chair and balancing without support. In this way, you're working toward increased balance, which is a skill you can cultivate with practice. The ability to balance is very important for us as we age so that we can avoid falls.

Of course, the breath is also very helpful in this practice. Try exhaling and sense energy moving down your body through the soles of your feet into the earth, and as you inhale, feel that energy moving up your body all the way to the top of your head.

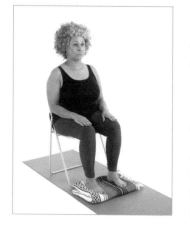

Chair Mountain Pose

From a chair: If standing is not possible, or if you feel unsteady when standing, Mountain Pose can be practiced in a chair. First decide if you have the core strength to sit up without leaning against the back of the chair. If so, sit slightly forward in the chair with your feet flat on the floor, directly under or slightly in front of your knees. If your feet don't easily reach the floor, use a folded blanket under them so that your knees are just below or level with your hips.

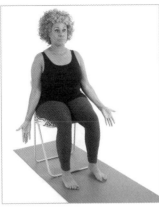

Chair Mountain Pose with Support

From a chair: If you have long legs, or a short chair, and your knees are higher than your hips, try putting a folded blanket on the seat of your chair.

Chair Mountain Pose Leaning Back

From a chair: If you need support to hold you up in this seated position, try scooting your buttocks all the way back in the chair. As you lean back, try to feel your spine lengthening upward. If you feel like you may fall out of the chair or are still unsteady, you can bring your feet farther forward or try placing a strap around your waist and the back of the chair like a seat belt.

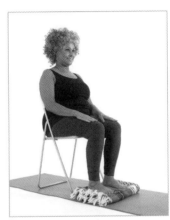

Once you're in chair Mountain Pose, try gently closing your eyes and focusing on your breath. Feel each exhalation grounding you down into the seat of the chair and through the soles of your feet. Each inhalation lifts and lengthens your spine all the way up through the top of your head.

SUPINE MOUNTAIN POSE

If you are practicing in bed, standing poses can be translated into supine poses that offer some of the same benefits. You can think of Corpse Pose as a bed variation of Mountain Pose and a great starting point for a bed or supine mat yoga practice.

Constructive Rest

From a bed or mat: To emphasize the grounding aspect of Mountain Pose while practicing in bed or lying on a mat, try practicing Constructive Rest. In this pose, your knees are bent with your feet placed slightly wider than your knees. Allow your knees to lean toward each other and hold each other up. Place your hands on your belly, or have your arms at your sides. Use a support under your neck if that's helpful. Focus on the grounding feeling of your hands on your belly and the soles of your feet against the floor or bed.

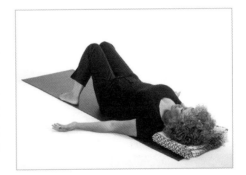

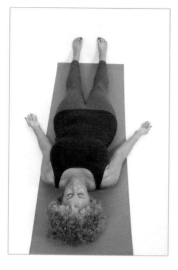

Supine Mountain Pose with Feet Press

From a bed or mat: Another way to practice supine Mountain Pose is to press the soles of your feet against a wall or the footboard of the bed. Focus on the pressure on the soles of your feet and use your breath to deepen that connection.

TREE POSE (VRKSASANA)

Tree Pose is a classic yoga practice that improves strength and balance and can be adapted in many ways. This pose is also a great place to explore the concept of grounding. Just as a tree can only send up tall branches when it has deep roots, you can learn how to ground down into the floor in order to lift and lengthen your body. Tree Pose also offers a hip-opening stretch, which is an element that can be emphasized or reduced in any of the following variations.

Many different arm positions can be used in this pose. Palms together at the chest may be the most gentle. More active positions include straight arms extended overhead in a Y shape or palms together overhead with the fingers interlaced and index fingers extended. In raised arm positions, be sure that your shoulders are relaxed down as your arms lift. Raised arms also offer an opportunity for shoulder strengthening. If you have high blood pressure, it's best to avoid holding your arms over your head for an extended period of time.

It's important that the supporting leg(s) in standing poses be engaged, so that the muscles are challenged and strengthened. Avoid locking the knee of the supporting leg, which can increase pressure on the joint and reduce the potential strengthening benefit of the practice.

In general, consciously engaging muscles while practicing can increase the strengthening benefits. But this needs to be done thoughtfully so that you're not simply increasing stress and tension in your body. As usual, yoga practice is about finding the balance between two extremes. The balance between flexibility and strength, and the balance between tension and relaxation.

Tree Pose with Back to Wall

From standing: To assist with balance, try standing with your back against the wall and your arms out to the sides with your palms against the wall. Begin by staring at a point on the floor or opposite wall. Bend your right

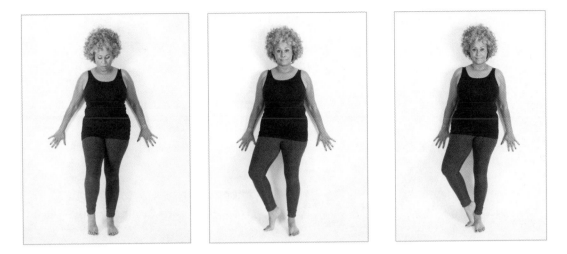

knee and place the toes of your right foot on the floor. Take a breath and find your balance. If this is comfortable, rotate your right knee out to the side. Then bring your right foot close to your left foot. Take a few breaths and then release. Repeat on the other side.

Tree Pose with Toes Down

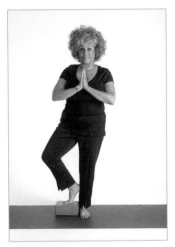

From standing: If you're practicing from a standing position, try placing the toes of your right leg on the floor with the heel resting against your left foot. Or rest your right foot on a block placed just on the inside of your left foot. If you're stable here, try raising your right foot a little higher up on your left leg. Use your breath to go deeper into the practice. Take a few breaths, and then switch sides.

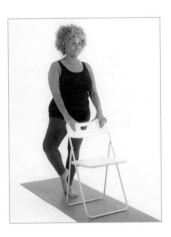

Tree Pose Holding a Chair

From standing: Stand behind a chair and hold on to the back. Another option is to turn so that you are standing behind the chair but perpendicular to it. Then you can hold the back of the chair with one hand, and engage the other arm in the pose.

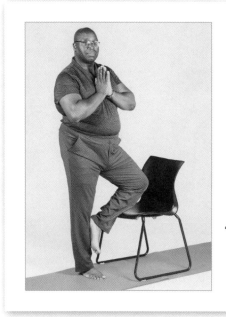

Michael Hayes:
Tree Pose with Chair Support

"Humor, patience, and self-compassion fuel the momentum of my practice. Balance, leverage, and weight are the three principles I use."

Chair Tree Pose

To practice Tree Pose while seated in a chair, consider what elements of the pose you can retain and what might be lost or reduced. In these variations, the element of balance is mostly removed, but you can still explore balance from a seated position, which might actually feel like a safer way to do it.

In a chair, you can explore balance by shifting your weight around and noticing how your body responds: what does it feel like to be completely balanced left and right, forward and back? What does it feel like to be unbalanced, like you might fall over? Exploring that sensation may help to overcome some of the fear that is often associated with standing balancing poses.

Similarly, the potential for strengthening the supporting leg is reduced in chair Tree Pose but not eliminated. To enhance it, try leaning forward while practicing this pose and consciously engaging the muscles of the supporting leg.

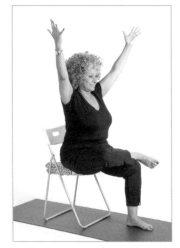

Chair Tree Pose with Crossed Leg

From a chair: Come to chair Mountain Pose. Place your right ankle on top of your left thigh, with your right knee out to the side. Your arms can be in any of the Tree Pose arm variations. If your leg is not comfortable in this position, try crossing your ankles instead.

Chair Tree Pose with Leg to Side

From a chair: Another variation, which emphasizes the hip-opening aspect of Tree Pose, can be done by placing a block on the outside of the right front leg of the chair. Ground into your left leg by leaning forward slightly, then bend your right knee and open that leg out to the side with your toes on the block. Bring your palms together at your chest.

Inhale and lengthen your arms overhead, in a Y shape, or out to the sides and bent at the elbows. Exhale as you feel energy moving down your left supporting leg and into your left foot. Inhale and feel length and lift through your body. Take a few breaths and release. Repeat on the other side.

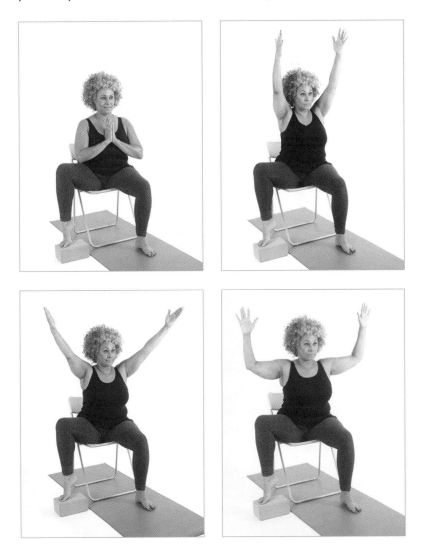

Bed Tree Pose

Tree Pose can also be practiced from a supine position. To experience the grounding quality of standing poses, it can be helpful to press your foot, or feet, into a wall or the footboard of the bed. A block between your foot and the wall or footboard can offer a softer more flexible surface to press into. Explore different arm and leg positions to find one that allows your body to feel grounded and open. The strengthening element may be reduced here, but you can add it by pressing your palms firmly together in front of your chest or raising your arms toward the ceiling.

Bed Tree Pose with Support

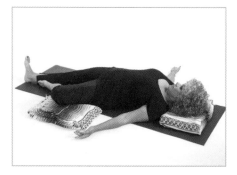

From a bed or mat: Press your right foot into the wall or footboard, if available. Bend your left leg and open your left knee out to the side. A folded blanket under your left knee can help keep your hips level and reduce the stretch on your left inner thigh. Bring your palms together at your chest and connect with your breath. Exhale down through your right foot, and inhale, sending energy up through your spine. Open your arms out to the sides, or find another comfortable arm position. Practice for few more breaths and then switch sides.

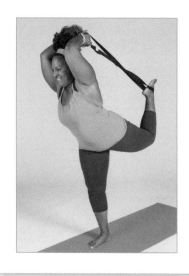

Dianne Bondy: King Dancer Pose with Strap

"This variation of King Dancer Pose lengthens my arms with the strap, because for me, reaching back behind me and trying to grab my foot is inaccessible. I love the strap because it makes my arms longer, and it gives me something to pull back on so I can find my balance. I believe props—props, props, props—are the gateway to accessibility. We need to look outside of the asana and look to props to help support, strengthen, lengthen, encourage, and embody our practice."

KING DANCER POSE (NATARAJASANA)

King Dancer Pose, like Tree Pose, offers many diverse benefits, including weight-bearing and balancing. It has the added benefit of stretching the hip flexors, particularly the psoas muscle, which is a deep core muscle that is often involved in lower back issues.

The psoas connects the legs to the torso and runs from the vertebrae in the lower back over the pelvis to the inner upper thigh. In fact, people who spend their days sitting may end up with shortened and tight psoas muscles. The psoas also contracts in the fight-or-flight response, so it is connected with trauma.

King Dancer Series Facing Wall

1. To help with balance, you can practice King Dancer Pose while facing a wall. Start in Mountain Pose about an arm's length from the wall, with the palm of your right hand flat on the wall. Bend your left knee, reach back with your left hand, and take hold of your left foot or ankle. Keep your left arm straight and feel like you're straightening your left leg to slowly bring the knee back.

2. If you can't comfortably reach your left foot or ankle, try placing a strap around your ankle and hold the strap in your hand.

3. If the position in step 1 or 2 feels comfortable, then try raising your right hand along the wall. If you feel balanced, you can lift your hand off the wall as you inhale. As you exhale, feel grounded through your

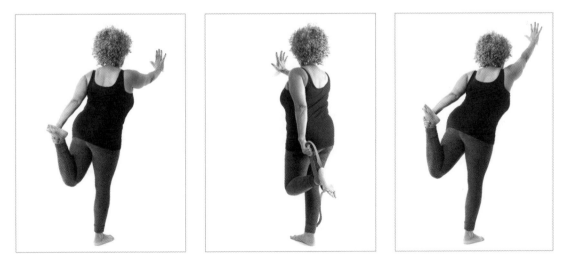

supporting leg, keeping the knee soft. Spot with your eyes. Take a few breaths and release. Repeat the practice on the other side.

King Dancer Pose with Foot on Chair

For more support, your raised foot can be placed on the seat of a chair behind you, and your hand can reach toward your foot without holding it.

Chair King Dancer Pose

The chair variation of King Dancer Pose offers a special challenge—finding a way to get hip extension (moving the knee back from the hip) in a seated position. In order to do this safely, you need to turn sideways in the chair. Keeping one hand on the back of the chair may help prevent you from falling off while practicing.

Chair King Dancer Pose Sitting Sideways

This is the same as the chair Warrior 1 Pose on page 89.

SIDE-LYING KING DANCER POSE

From a bed or mat: You can practice King Dancer Pose on the floor or in bed by lying on your side. Lie on your right side and bend both knees. Place a folded blanket under your head so your neck is neutral. Reach back with your left hand to try to take hold of your left ankle. A support can be placed under your left leg if that feels more stable. Reach your right arm forward along the floor. Inhale and feel like you're straightening your left leg; exhale and feel grounded and supported by the floor.

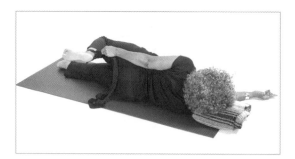

Eagle Pose (Garudasana)

Eagle Pose is a standing balancing pose that incorporates crossing the arms and legs, actions that cross the midline of the body and are helpful for increasing communication between the right and left hemispheres of the brain.

Eagle Pose with Back to Wall and Block

From standing: To support your balance in Eagle Pose, you can use the wall and a block. Begin by standing with your back to the wall but just slightly away from it. Place the block on the outside of your left foot. Stare at a spot in front of you. Bend your knees to allow your back to press into the wall for support.

Lift your right leg and cross it over the left, bringing the toes of your right foot to the block. Hug yourself with your arms. Inhale and lengthen your spine. Exhale and ground down into your left foot. If this is comfortable, you can lift your hands slowly, bringing the backs of them together. Or have the back of one hand against the outside of your opposite elbow.

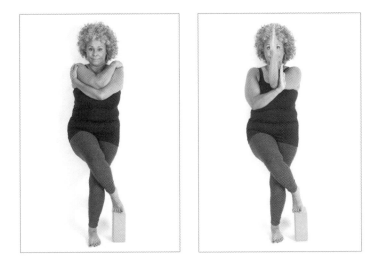

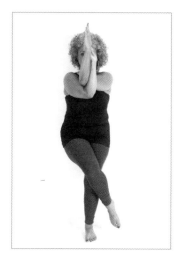

Eagle Pose with Back to Wall

From standing: You can also practice Eagle Pose with your back to the wall but without a block under the raised foot.

Chair Eagle Pose Series

From a chair: Starting in chair Mountain Pose, cross your right leg over the left, or cross your right ankle over your left. Bend your right arm and bring your left arm underneath it, holding gently. If this is comfortable, reach around with the left hand to try and bring the backs of the hands together.

If this is too challenging, try giving yourself a hug with both hands on opposite shoulders. Or hold your hands together with a strap. Use your breath to help ground yourself into the floor by leaning forward slightly and pressing your right foot firmly into the floor. Take a few breaths, then practice on the other side.

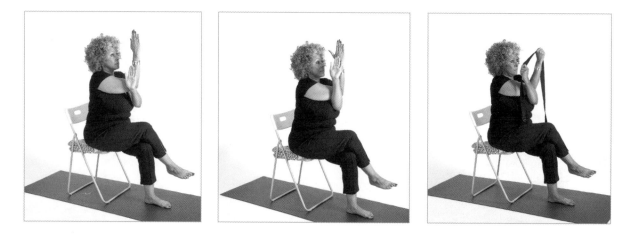

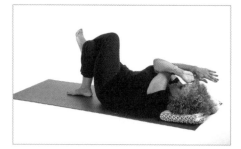

BED EAGLE POSE

From a bed: Start in bed Mountain Pose (Corpse Pose), bend your knees, and place your feet flat on the floor or bed. Cross your left leg over the right, or cross your ankles if you prefer. Give yourself a hug, with your hands holding opposite shoulders. If this is comfortable, lift your arms in front of your body and wrap one arm under the other. (It doesn't matter which is on top as long as you switch arms when you practice on the other side.) Press your right foot firmly into the floor or bed.

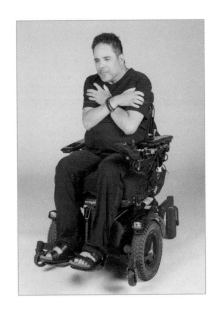

Chris Stigas:
Eagle Pose with Hug

"For me, my breathing and lungs make up a lot of my core stability. When I am exhaling out in this pose, I lose that characteristic. This makes me have to rebalance myself using other minor muscles outside of my breathing stability system. It forces me to engage these core muscles for balance, and it really requires quite a bit of focus and concentration where I can find that alternative new point of stability and balance."

Mat Eagle Pose

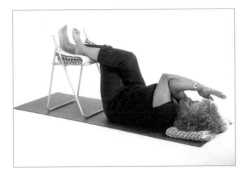

From a mat: Similar to the bed Eagle Pose, you can practice Eagle Pose while lying on your mat with a chair under your legs. Press your legs into the seat of the chair to create the sensation of grounding, and use any Eagle Pose arm position that is comfortable for you.

WARRIOR 1 AND 2 POSE (VIRABHADRASANA I AND II)

Warrior 1 Pose is a standing lunge with raised arms. Warrior 2 Pose offers a different type of lunge where the front leg is bent. Both poses stretch the deep muscles of the pelvis, hips, and lower back. They are great poses for reclaiming power and strength.

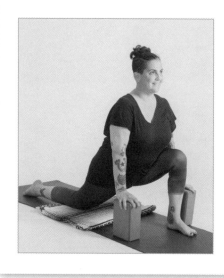

Sarit Rogers:
Raised Lunge with Blocks

"The raised lunge helps inform a different awareness of my hips and pelvic girdle. Because I practice with fibromyalgia and also have degenerative disc disease in my lumbar and arthritis in my sacroiliac (SI) joint, creating stability is key. It's easy for me to dump into my low back, which often feels good, but the impact is negative later. I work intimately with intention versus impact in my personal practice so that I can truly honor my experience and nurture healing rather than promoting performance."

Chair Lunge

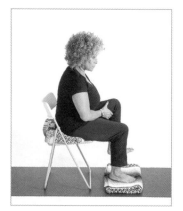

From a chair: Start in chair Mountain Pose. Keep your back long, and ground with your right foot while lifting your left leg up, hugging your left knee to your chest. You can hold your leg under the thigh as you raise it toward your abdomen.

SUPINE KNEE TO CHEST

From a bed or mat: Lie on your back with your legs extended out in front of you. Bend your right knee and hold the back of your right thigh. Hug your knee toward your chest. Hold for a few breaths, or come in and out of the pose with your breath. Practice on the other side.

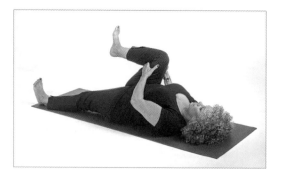

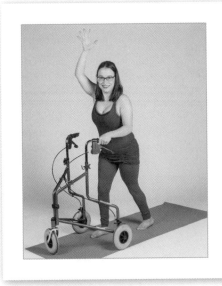

**Elizabeth Wojtowicz:
Warrior 1 Pose with Support**

"It helps to really just open my body, and with cerebral palsy my body is super tight, so poses that help to elongate my body feel really good. What yoga is for me is about accessibility and community."

CHAIR WARRIOR 1 POSE

From a chair: You can do Warrior 1 Pose in a chair by sitting sideways. Turn to the right, and move forward in the seat so the left side of your buttocks comes off the chair. Be sure that you're stable, and hold the back of the chair with your right hand for security. Press your left leg back to feel a stretch on the front of that hip. You can place a bolster or block under your left knee for additional support. Exhale and ground down into the chair and your left knee. Inhale and raise your left arm over your head. Hold for a few breaths and then switch sides.

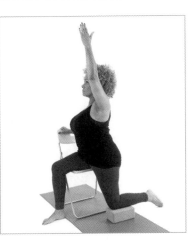

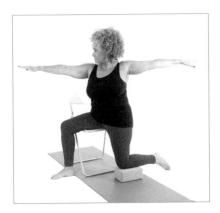

CHAIR WARRIOR 2 POSE

From a chair: Bring your legs into the same position as for chair Warrior 1 Pose. If you feel stable in the chair, extend both arms out at shoulder height. Point your right arm forward and your left arm back. Inhale and lengthen your spine; exhale and ground into your right foot, left knee, and sit bones.

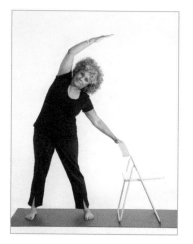

SIDE BEND

Standing Side Bend with Chair

From standing: Stand sideways behind a chair, and gently hold on to the back with your left hand for support. Widen your legs to a stable distance. Inhale, raise your right arm over your head, and lengthen your spine. Exhale, bending toward the chair and lengthen the right side of your body. Keep your neck neutral. Hold for a breath or two and release. Repeat on the opposite side.

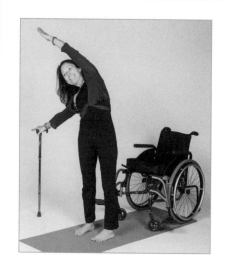

Cherie Hotchkiss:
Side Bend with Support

"My assistive devices are a natural extension of my body now and are essential to maintaining my independence and mobility. They even create access to physical poses in my yoga practice, just as using traditional yoga props help all differently abled bodies."

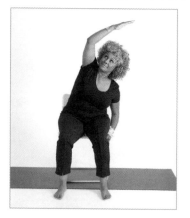

Chair Side Bend

From a chair: Sit in chair Mountain Pose. Hold the seat of the chair with your left hand for support. Inhale, raise your right arm over your head, and lengthen your spine. Exhale and bend to the left. Keep your neck neutral. Hold for a breath or two and release. Repeat on the other side.

Lying Side Bend

From a bed or mat: Lying on your back, cross your left ankle over your right and raise your arms over your head. Take hold of your left wrist with your right hand. Inhale, lengthen your spine, and bend toward the right, gently stretching the left side of your body. Hold for a breath or two and release. Repeat on the other side.

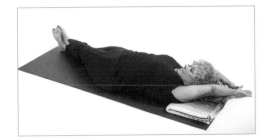

Side-Lying Side Bend

From a bed or mat: Lie on your left side with a bolster under your ribcage. Bend your left knee for balance. Raise your arms over your head and place a blanket between your head and left arm to keep your neck neutral. Inhale and lengthen your spine as you stretch the right side of your body by reaching your right arm and right leg in opposite directions. Hold for a breath or two and release. Repeat on the other side.

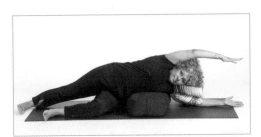

BACKWARD BENDING 7

OUR POSTURE can be a reflection of our current state of mind as well as our past experiences. Slouching may reflect how we feel immediately after receiving some bad news, or it may reflect years of sitting at a desk using a computer. Asana practice, and in particular backward bending poses, can assist us in undoing some of our long-term postural habits.

Posture is also crafted by the universal forces of gravity and time. As we age, the spine tends to become kyphotic, or rounded in the upper back. This can have grave implications for other systems in the body as well as our general health. For example, a rounded upper back can mean reduced flexibility of the ribs and decreased space for the lungs to expand as we inhale.[1]

Backward bending poses create extension and space in the spine, although postural issues that are genetic or have developed over a lifetime can be slow to change, if they do so at all. Many people need variations to the traditional backward bending poses to practice in a safe and gentle way.

COBRA POSE (BHUJANGASANA)/SPHINX POSE (SALAMBA BHUJANGASANA)

Cobra Pose is one of the most effective poses for creating spinal extension, expanding the chest, lengthening the neck, and strengthening the upper back. To benefit the upper back, it can be more useful to practice an Accessible Cobra Pose, focusing on using the back muscles to lift the chest as high as is comfortable without pressing into the hands.

When the arms are extended in front of the shoulders, the pose is usually referred to as Sphinx Pose. Some people find that Sphinx Pose releases their lower back, while others may feel that it increases pressure in that area.

Here are the main benefits of Cobra Pose and Sphinx Pose:

- Improving posture and expanding the chest
- Energizing
- Massaging the abdominal organs

Can you find these benefits in the variation that works best for your body?

Accessible Cobra Pose

From a mat: It can be helpful to place a folded blanket underneath your pelvis when practicing Cobra Pose to avoid pressure or pinching in your lower back. The blanket tilts your pelvis posteriorly and lengthens your lower back, which reduces the lumbar lordosis (the lower back curve).

Lie on your abdomen with your palms on the floor under your shoulders. As you come into the pose, exhale and press your tailbone toward the floor; as you inhale, slowly lengthen your spine and lift your head, neck, and chest.

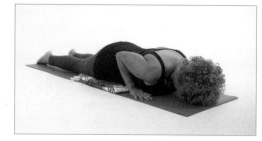 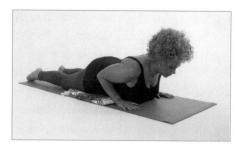

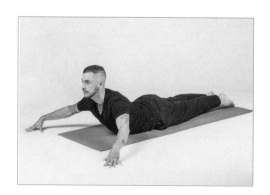

Tobias Wiggins:
Sphinx Pose with Wide Arms

"Doing mental health work with the queer community has helped expand my knowledge of how trauma and emotional blockages can be stored in the body. Backbends tend to be the master-opener of these raw emotions, as they specifically target energy channels that travel up through the spine. When I backbend, I practice finding trust in myself as I advance toward the unknown.

For queer people—who face disproportionate amounts of rejection from family and friends, violence, and systemic injustice—this foundation of trust may feel more precarious. Sphinx Pose, or Salamba Bhujuangasana, is a gentle backbend and chest opener that can be done actively or passively. Not only does it sooth the nervous system, but it also employs the forearms for support (*salamba* = "with support"), a somatic reminder that we can always return to our personal support system. As a queer and transgender person, this embodied reminder has been especially helpful to me for healing and building resilience."

Try to use your upper back muscles rather than pressing into your hands, and keep the focus in your upper back rather than coming up higher. Take a few breaths, then come down as slowly as you came up.

Cobra Pose with Head Down

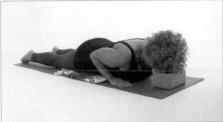

From a mat: If you have kyphosis (rounded upper back), then it may be safer to keep your head in line with your upper spine and not allow your neck to go into extension. To assist with keeping your head down, you can rest your forehead on a block at a height that feels comfortable for your neck, where it's lengthening without bending back.

Cobra Pose with Chest Support

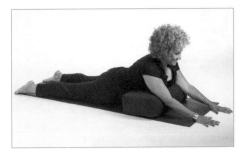

From a mat: For some people, placing a bolster or blanket under the chest helps to support the upper body in Cobra Pose. Experiment with blankets and bolsters of different heights to see what feels comfortable for you. Also, experiment with the location of the support so that it helps to expand your chest rather than making it feel compressed.

Kneeling Cobra Pose

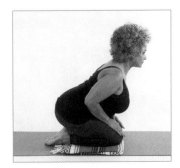

From kneeling: If you aren't able to lie flat on your abdomen, you can practice Cobra Pose from a kneeling position. This also protects your neck from too much extension. Sit on your heels on a folded blanket and hinge forward from the hips with your hands on your thighs. Keep your back long and bend your head down as you exhale. Then inhale and lengthen your spine, raising your head, neck, and chest, just as you would on the floor. Keep your focus in your upper back. Take a few breaths and then release.

Standing Cobra Pose

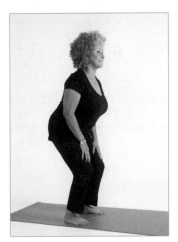

From standing: Similarly, Cobra Pose can be done in a standing position, which also avoids pressure on the front of the body. Begin in Mountain Pose. Bend your knees and place your hands on your thighs for support. Lower your head down as you exhale. Inhale and slowly curl up your head, neck, and upper chest. Be careful not to drop your head back too far; keep your neck long. Take a few breaths and release.

Wall Cobra Pose

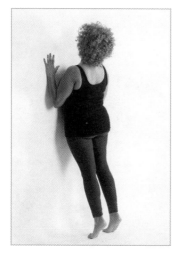

From standing: Try to use the wall the way you might use the floor. Stand facing and a few inches away from the wall in Mountain Pose. Place your hands on the wall at shoulder height. Exhale and lean toward the wall. As you inhale, lengthen your spine and try pulling your hands toward the floor. Raise your chin and lift up onto your toes to get the feeling of length in your spine. Be sure not to bring your head too far back. Instead, focus on lengthening your neck. Take a few breaths and slowly come down.

Chair Cobra Pose

Chair Cobra Pose is an effective part of a chair yoga routine because of the postural benefits. The challenge is finding a way to practice in the chair without allowing your head to fall too far backward, since that can lead to compression of the nerves and arteries in the back of your neck. Be particularly careful with head movements if you have osteoporosis in your neck.

Chair Cobra Pose with Arms Back

From a chair: From chair Mountain Pose, bring your hands to the back of the chair, down toward the seat. Lean forward and slowly lift your head as you inhale. Feel your chest moving forward and your spine lengthening in your upper back.

Chair Cobra Pose with Hands Up

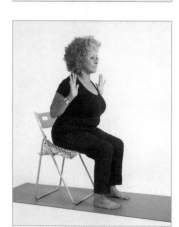

From a chair: You can practice chair Cobra Pose with your hands in front of your shoulders, palms forward. This is similar to Accessible Cobra Pose on the mat, which can help to move your shoulders down and back.

Chair Cobra Pose with Bolster

From a chair: To add an abdominal massage, try practicing chair Cobra Pose with a bolster on your lap. Place your arms over the bolster to hold it snugly against your belly. Exhale and bend forward over the bolster, gently lowering your head. As you inhale, lengthen your neck and slowly lift your head, neck, and upper chest. Keep your shoulders back and gently pull the bolster toward your belly, which can help lengthen your spine even more. Hold for

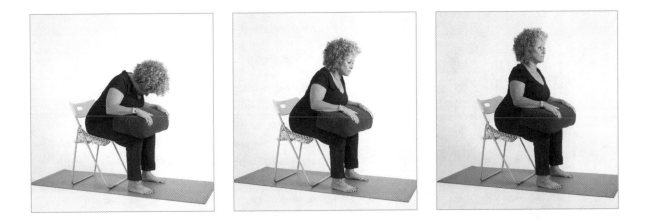

a few breaths and then slowly lower back down, reversing the movements you used to come into the pose.

FISH POSE (MATSYASANA)

It's also possible to work on expanding the chest and improving posture from a supine position by practicing a variation of Fish Pose.

Accessible Fish Pose

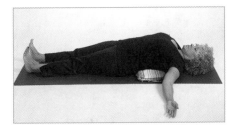

From a bed or mat: Place a folded blanket or small bolster under your upper back and lie back over it with your arms out to the sides. You can experiment with the placement of the blanket to see what feels best for you. You may want to try it under the back of your ribs to help expand your lungs and improve posture.

Fish Pose with Bolster

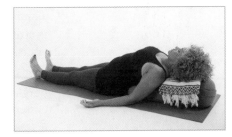

From a bed or mat: You can also use a larger bolster or higher support. Try to have the end of the bolster at the bottom of your ribcage. In this case, you may need an additional blanket under your neck. While in the pose, take advantage of your expanded ribcage to do some deep breathing. You can rest in this position for a few minutes, if it is comfortable.

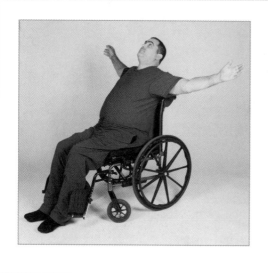

Rudra Swartz:
Chair Fish Pose

"When I first started practicing yoga after using a wheelchair, backbends were my favorite poses. At first I would put my forearms on my armrests and my feet on the floor and bend way backward. After this asana, I would sit up and it would seem like my mind was the most restful it had been all day. After learning more backbends in the wheelchair, I started to use the bolster when I couldn't necessarily lift myself up on my armrests. I found bending backward over the bolster behind my back very powerful."

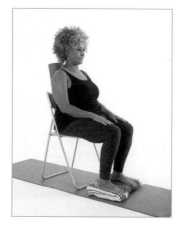

Chair Fish Pose

From a chair: Place a rolled yoga mat behind your back to press into. This support can help to expand your chest and improve posture. Roll the mat loosely to make it a little softer, and place it so it reaches from the bottom of your rib cage up to your head. You could also use a folded blanket behind your upper back with the chair against a wall.

LOCUST POSE (SALABHASANA)

Recently, researchers at Boston Medical Center showed that yoga was as good as physical therapy for treating lower back pain, which is one of the most common causes of disability in the United States.[2] This research demonstrates what yoga practitioners have long known—that yoga can help to strengthen and align the back.

Of course, yoga can also exacerbate or cause low back injuries if not practiced correctly, which is why it is so important for yoga practitioners with lower back concerns to practice very slowly and with care. Locust Pose is a powerful practice for strengthening the back that may not be accessible for many of us. Even Half Locust Pose (Ardha Salabhasana) can be too challenging if you are new to yoga or have lower back issues.

Traditionally, Locust Pose is done by lying on your abdomen with your arms tucked under your body. Either both legs are raised, or one leg is raised in Half Locust Pose. The practice can also be done with your arms alongside your body and your arms coming up when your legs come up.

The main benefit of practicing Locust Pose is increasing flexibility and strength in the lower back, buttocks, and hips. To achieve this, try using a blanket under the front of your pelvis, as described earlier for Accessible Cobra Pose. In this variation, you can keep your arms alongside your body, which can also be more comfortable if you have wrist pain or arthritis in your hands.

Half Locust Pose with Toes Down

From a mat: Half Locust Pose can be practiced by keeping the toes of your extended leg on the floor. Instead of lifting your entire leg, you lift the knee and the leg is lengthened through the heel.

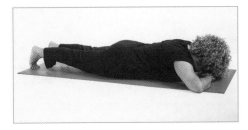

Half Locust Pose with Support

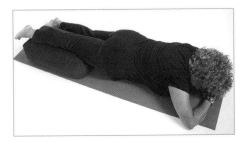

From a mat: Half Locust Pose can be done with a bolster or blanket under one leg to hold it up. Try to create length in the lifted leg, and try to avoid twisting your lower back and SI joint.

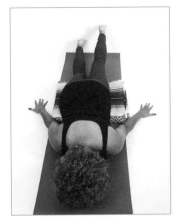

Locust Pose with Feet on Wall

From a mat: To come up higher in Locust Pose or Half Locust Pose, try practicing with your feet against a wall. You can carefully allow your feet to climb the wall behind you. Be sure not to strain in this pose by walking your feet up too high.

Standing Half Locust Pose

From standing: If lying on your abdomen is uncomfortable, you can practice Half Locust Pose from a standing position facing a wall or holding on to the back of a chair. The challenge in standing Locust Pose is to keep your torso upright and not hinge forward at the hips. With your upper body steady, inhale and lengthen your right leg out behind you, resting on the toes of your right foot. If this is comfortable, you can raise your leg higher. Once again check that your torso isn't moving forward. Take a breath and release. You can repeat a few times on each side.

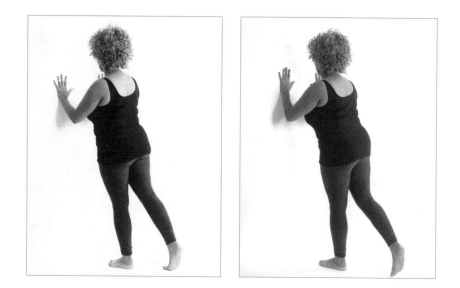

FORWARD BENDING 8

COMMON SENSE tells us that relaxation is simply the absence of stress, but it's not so simple. Relaxation can be actively cultivated by stimulating the parasympathetic nervous system (PNS), and yoga's ability to do so may be the main reason why it is so powerful. Yoga really is an antidote to our stressed-out modern lives.

The PNS is the rest-and-digest, down-regulating aspect of our autonomic nervous system (the part of the nervous system we usually don't control). Through yoga, we can find ways to stimulate the PNS and actively relax. "Parasympathetic stimulation" may seem like an oxymoron, but that's exactly what we're doing. In particular, slow breathing, relaxation techniques, and meditation can support the PNS.

Through experience, yogis have also found that forward bending stimulates the PNS. By folding forward, we calm the nervous system as we literally connect with ourselves and turn within. We also create a safe feeling position where the sensitive front of the body is well protected. This inward energetic experience is the mark of forward bending and one of its most profound benefits.

However, for many of us, the standard forward bending postures are not accessible because of lower back issues and a variety of other reasons. These issues often stem from, or contribute to, tight hamstring, hip, and buttock muscles. Forward bending can address much of the tightness in these areas, but there is a fine line between stretching and straining in these poses. Ironically, the very poses that can release tension in these sensitive areas can also cause injury if practiced too aggressively.

BENDING FORWARD SAFELY

One of the most important things to learn when practicing forward bends is how to hinge from the hip joint rather than rounding the lower back to bend forward. This rounding movement is known as loaded flexion, and it is such a large source of injury that many workplaces have put up posters explaining how to avoid it: "Lift with the legs, not with the back." Ultimately, all movement is healthy, but for those of us with lower back injuries, osteoporosis, and arthritis, it's especially important to learn how to bend forward without loaded flexion.

Translated into asana practice, this means that we need to work on releasing the hamstrings so that the hips can rotate and the top of the pelvis is free to move forward. The issue is that the hamstrings originate at the sit bones, and when they are tight, they pull down on those bones and prevent pelvic rotation. This forces the forward bending movement higher, into the vertebrae of the lower back. The lower back can be stretched gently, but with too much force, injuries such as pulled muscles and slipped or herniated discs can occur.

The SI joint, where the sacrum connects to the pelvis, is another area in the lower back where injury can occur in forward bends, especially in asymmetrical poses like Head to Knee Pose (Janu Sirsasana).

An effective way to practice seated forward bends is to consider two approaches to the same pose: one focusing on the hamstring stretch and another variation focusing on the inward experience. In the first approach, only hinge forward to the point where you can still keep your spine (including your neck) neutral and elongated. Focus on hip rotation and lengthening the back of your legs. In this approach, it may be helpful to place a strap around the ball(s) of the foot (or feet) of the extended leg(s) and hold one side of the strap in each hand. This is especially useful if you have very tight hamstrings or a back injury, which can make rounding the back risky.

The second approach is to hinge forward into the pose, as described earlier. Then once you come to the point where can you no longer maintain neutral, gradually release your spine forward into an evenly distributed curve, relaxing your head down or releasing your hamstrings by bending your knees before coming forward. This approach focuses on gently stretching the lower back and the back of the neck, which stimulates the PNS and allows for a quieting of the nervous system and, in turn, the mind.

The main benefits of forward bending are:

- Stretching the hamstrings and back of the body
- Calming anxiety, going inward, soothing stress

Accessible Head to Knee Pose

From a mat: Sit with your legs stretched out in front of you. Bend your left knee and rotate it out to the side. You can place a blanket under the knee for support. Notice if you're comfortable sitting on the floor with your right leg extended out in front of you. If you find you're leaning back in this position or using your abdominal muscles or hands to help hold you up, then it's a good idea to find a way to adapt the posture.

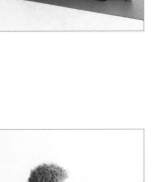

To do this you need to release the stretch in your hamstrings and find more length in your spine. The most effective way is to bend your right knee and place a support underneath it. Or, to encourage hip rotation and the forward movement of the top of your pelvis, you can sit on a folded blanket. It's also helpful to use a strap to connect to your feet without straining to touch your toes.

Inhale as you lengthen your spine, and exhale as you hinge forward at your hips with a long spine just until you feel a stretch in the back of your right leg; stop there. On the next exhalation, you can relax your head and shoulders, if that feels comfortable. Try to avoid rounding your back. Take a few breaths here, then lengthen your spine as you inhale to come up. Repeat on the other side.

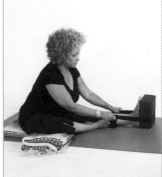

Head to Knee Pose with Foot Support

From a mat: If you have a dropped foot or weakness in the lower leg, you can place your foot against a wall or on a block that is held in place with a strap. This aligns your foot and leg, while also providing a surface to gently press against.

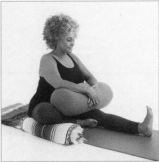

Head to Knee Pose with Bolster

From a mat: To encourage lifting and lengthening your spine, try placing a bolster on your lap. Rather than reaching toward your foot in the forward bend, try to press into the bolster with your arms as you lift your torso. You can place the bolster on and parallel to the extended leg. Or you can position it perpendicular to the extended leg and close to your abdomen.

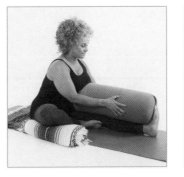

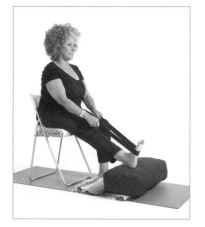
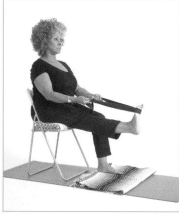

Chair Head to Knee Pose

From a chair: Sit toward the front of the seat, but be sure that you aren't going to fall out. You can rest the foot of your extended leg on a bolster or block with a strap around the ball of the foot. Hold the ends of the strap in your hands, and use the tension to help lift and lengthen your spine as you inhale. Exhale and hinge forward until you feel a stretch on the back of your leg without rounding your back. Hold for a few breaths, then switch sides. This can also be done by keeping your raised foot in the air instead of resting it on a bolster.

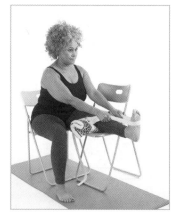

Chair Head to Knee Pose with Second Chair

From a chair: You can also practice by placing your extended leg on a second chair. Be sure that the back of your knee is on the seat of that chair so that your knee does not hyperextend. You can turn the second chair sideways and place it as close to your chair as possible. A strap around the ball of your foot can be used to add extra support and to encourage lengthening in your spine, rather than rounding in your back, as you bend forward.

Hand to Big Toe Pose (Supta Padangusthasana)

To avoid loaded flexion and rounding your spine in forward bends, you can practice Hand to Big Toe Pose. This is very similar to seated forward bends, but in this position the body has a different relationship to gravity. In this supine forward bend the spine is completely supported, so the focus can be on the back of the leg. Using a strap can be very helpful to control the stretch and create structure in the pose. You can practice with your arms straight or bent, holding the strap in a relaxed way. Or try one of the strap variations that follow.

Hand to Big Toe Pose with Strap Variations

Straight Arms

From a bed or mat: Lie on your back with both knees bent. Place a strap around the ball of your right foot and lengthen that foot toward the ceiling. Try to keep your arms straight and hold the strap close to your foot. If it's more comfortable, you can place a folded blanket under your head. Focus on the stretch in the back of your right leg. Inhale as you lengthen your leg, and exhale as you try to relax the muscles in the back of your leg. Take a few breaths and then release. Repeat the practice on the other side.

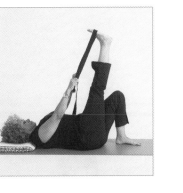

Bent Arms

In this variation, you bend your arms and rest the tops of your arms alongside your body. You can keep your left knee bent or extended out on the floor, which can help to keep your back neutral and encourage you not to lift your tailbone off the floor.

Arms Overhead

To emphasize lengthening the back of your leg, and to avoid gripping the strap too tightly with your hands, you can make a large loop with the strap. Place one side around the ball of your right foot or the back of your right ankle, and hold the other side in your hands. Put your palms together with thumbs extended, as you straighten your arms and raise them toward the ceiling. You can hold the strap with your thumbs.

Handles

Similarly, with the strap in a large loop, place the middle of the loop around your right foot. Then allow the two ends to hang down and place your hands in the loops, using them like handles. This can be helpful if you want to avoid gripping the strap with your hands, or if you have arthritis in your hands.

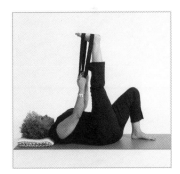

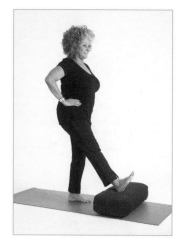

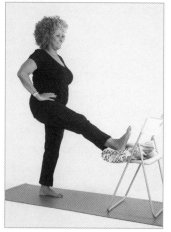

Standing Hand to Big Toe Pose

From standing: This pose is a variation of Extended Hand to Big Toe Pose (Utthita Hasta Padangusthasana). The added element of balancing on one foot can make this a challenging and fun pose. Begin in Mountain Pose with a bolster on the floor in front of you. To assist with balance, focus your eyes on one spot. Shift your weight to your left leg, keeping the knee soft and the muscles of the leg engaged. Raise your right leg and place your heel on the bolster, keeping your leg straight.

Your hands can be on your hips, or you can use a strap to connect to your raised foot. If you prefer, you can also practice with your raised leg on the seat of a chair. Make sure that you are well balanced and won't fall over. Hold for a few breaths, then switch legs.

Seated Forward Bend (Paschimottanasana)

In Seated Forward Bend, both legs are extended out in front of you. This can be more intense than bending over one leg at a time. But the symmetry of the pose can support those who have lower back injuries, in particular SI joint issues. Most of the variations used in Head to Knee Pose also apply to this pose, and here are a few additional ideas to make the practice more accessible.

Accessible Seated Forward Bend

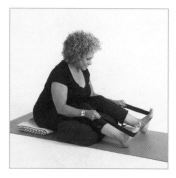

From a mat: You can do Seated Forward Bend sitting on the floor with a bolster under both knees. Hinging forward at your hips, keep your spine long and allow your arms to rest alongside your body without reaching toward your toes. Or use a strap looped around your feet to help keep your spine long by pulling gently and using the tension to lift and lengthen your torso.

Seated Forward Bend with Blocks

From a mat: One thing to avoid in a Seated Forward Bend is straining to reach your toes. It's human nature to want to touch your toes, but it can be counterproductive in a forward bend. Instead, try to focus on lengthening your spine. To help with this, try placing one block on each side of your extended legs. Rather than reach toward your toes, rest your hands on top of the blocks. Try to press into the blocks to engage your core muscles, lifting from your inner body. Be especially patient in forward bending, and spend more time releasing and relaxing in the pose rather than trying to get somewhere. Pay attention to your breath, and be sure it's smooth and relaxed.

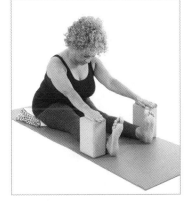

Seated Forward Bend with Hugging Legs

From a mat: You can also try bending your knees deeply and hugging your legs toward your chest with your arms under your thighs. Inhale and lengthen your spine, and exhale as you relax forward.

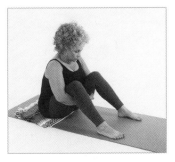

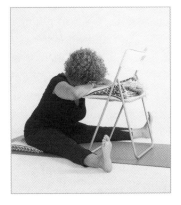

Seated Forward Bend with Head on Chair

From a mat: Sit on the floor with a chair facing you. Your legs can be under the chair or on either side of it. Inhale and lengthen your spine; exhale and hinge forward from your hips until you can rest your arms and head on the seat of the chair. Notice how a gentle pressure on your forehead can be soothing to the nervous system. Or try pressing into the seat to lift and lengthen your spine.

Chair Seated Forward Bend

From a chair: Extend both legs in front of you and rest both feet on a bolster or the floor. Use a strap around both feet, if that feels safe. Be careful not to fall out of the chair. As you inhale, lengthen your spine; as you exhale, hinge forward at your hips just until you feel a stretch in the backs of your legs.

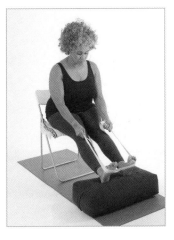

SEATED WIDE-ANGLE POSE (UPAVISTHA KONASANA)

Seated Wide-Angle Pose provides a forward bend with an added inner thigh stretch. Similar to other seated forward bends, the focus is on hip rotation. Sit with your legs wide apart. To make the pose more accessible, you can bend your knees to release your hamstrings. Inhale and lengthen your spine. As you exhale, hinge forward from your hips, keeping your spine long. You can rest your hands on your legs or the floor in front of you, or bring your hands alongside or behind you if you feel like you're leaning back. Take a few breaths and then release.

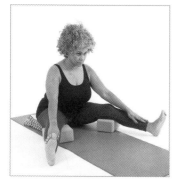

Accessible Seated Wide-Angle Pose

From a mat: You can practice Seated Wide-Angle Pose with blankets or blocks under both knees. Keep your spine long, and don't strain to touch your toes.

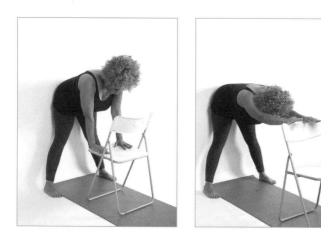

Standing Wide-Angle Pose

From standing: Another way to practice Wide-Angle Pose is standing with your buttocks against the wall and a chair in front of you. Place your hands or forearms on the seat of the chair, or move the chair farther away and extend your arms to hold on to the back. Your feet are parallel and wide apart. In this pose, gravity assists the lengthening of your hamstrings and the release of the back of your neck.

Wide-Angle Inversion

From a mat: From Legs-Up-the-Wall Pose, you can separate your legs and allow gravity to help them open. As with Hand to Big Toe Pose, this variation allows for a stretch to the hamstrings and inner thighs while keeping the spine supported and relaxed.

PIGEON POSE (KAPOTASANA)

Pigeon Pose is generally considered a backward bend. But in these adapted forms it's more of a forward bend that focuses on stretching the hip. In general, the hip area only needs mild stretching. But many advanced yoga poses force the hip outside the normal range of motion, which is unhealthy for the joint in the long run. Practice Pigeon Pose with gentleness and sensitivity, focusing on the calming, inward quality that a hip stretch and a gentle forward bend can bring.

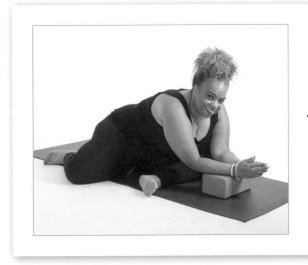

Natalie Dunbar:
Pigeon Pose with Bent Leg

"I am fuller in my midbody, and I tend to get uncomfortable when I have to fold forward over my abundance, so in putting the block in front of me and bending the back leg, I have more accessibility and more stability. I'm aligned a little bit better, and I'm able to bring the floor up to me so that the pose is more accessible."

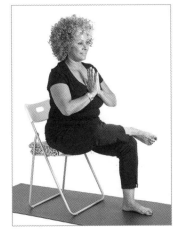

Chair Pigeon Pose

From a chair: Pigeon Pose can be done by sitting in chair Mountain Pose and resting one ankle on the opposite knee. Bring your palms together at your chest. Sit tall and begin to hinge slightly forward until you start to feel a stretch in the hip of your raised leg. Take a few breaths there, then switch sides.

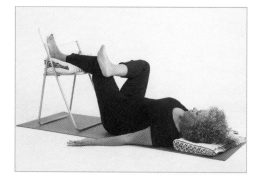

Supine Pigeon Pose

From a bed or mat: Lie in Savasana with both knees bent. Raise your right foot onto your left thigh with your right knee stretching away from your torso. Rest here if you already feel a stretch in your right hip. If this is comfortable, take hold of your left thigh and pull your legs gently closer to your torso. If you're practicing on a mat, you can rest your feet on a chair to begin.

INVERTING 9

IN MANY WAYS, the practice of yoga is about changing your perspective, shifting your relationship with your body as well as your mind. As you change your perspective, you may begin to see your body in a new light—as the essential vehicle for your temporary human journey. Instead of idolizing or demonizing it, you can treat it with love.

Practices like inversions help us to make this shift by literally turning the body on its head. Full inversions are defined as those that bring the heart over the head. With this new relationship between heart and head, the mind gets quieter and allows space for the wisdom of the heart to speak, connecting back to the goal of yoga: calm the mind, free the heart.

Bringing the head below the heart offers a variety of other benefits, including resting the heart and lowering blood pressure. The heart first feeds itself, bringing oxygenated blood through the coronary arteries; then it focuses on bringing blood to the brain. To do this, your blood pressure is constantly adapting to your position in relation to gravity to regulate how much blood is getting to your brain.

This is why it's important to make slow transitions from supine to seated to standing poses when practicing. If you stand up too quickly, it may take a moment for your blood pressure to compensate, and you may experience lightheadedness or dizziness. This is especially true for seniors and those with compromised cardiovascular systems.

Inversions, like so many yoga practices, support the body in weathering the eternal forces of gravity and time. Many of the challenges associated with aging are specifically related to gravity: postural issues, prolapsed organs, varicose veins, hemorrhoids, and more. The issue is that inversions are often physically challenging postures that put pressure on the head and neck. For many people, poses like Headstand (Sirsasana) and Shoulderstand (Sarvangasana) are not accessible.

If you can't do these full inversions, there are many benefits to practicing variations of these poses that are gentler or where the head isn't below the heart, and only part of the body is inverted. For example, inverting an arm by raising it can improve lymph drainage in that arm. Let's explore a variety of accessible inversions to gain access to some of the benefits of turning the body on its head—without literally having to do that!

DOWNWARD-FACING DOG POSE (ADHO MUKHA SVANASANA)

Downward-Facing Dog Pose may be the quintessential yoga practice, but most people don't think of it as an inversion. In fact, the pose is quite complicated and incorporates many different dynamics, including forward bending (hip flexion) and inversion. One special quality of this pose is that there is no weight on the head or neck, and since the feet remain on the floor, it doesn't demand the level of balance that so many other inversions do. Downward-Facing Dog Pose offers an inversion to the upper body, including changing the relationship between head and heart, while keeping the lower body grounded. But there are some contraindications to having the head below the heart. This includes glaucoma or any inflammation in the head.

There are many variations of Downward-Facing Dog Pose that offer some of the same benefits but in a more accessible fashion. Here are a few essential elements of the pose that you can explore. Can you find one or more of these elements in the form that you practice?

- Inverting the upper body
- Stretching the backs of the legs (calves and hamstrings), arms, and armpit area
- Safe forward bending (hip flexion as opposed to spinal flexion, which is discussed in chapter 8)
- Creating traction in the spine (lengthening without compression)
- Strengthening the arms and shoulders

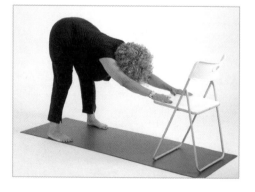

Downward-Facing Dog Pose with Hands on Chair

From standing: You can experience Downward-Facing Dog Pose without bringing your hands to the floor by placing them on a chair instead. Stand in Mountain Pose with a chair about three feet in front of you, or whatever distance feels right for your body. Soften your knees and hinge forward at your hips, reaching out for the back or seat of the chair. Use whichever is at the most comfortable height for you.

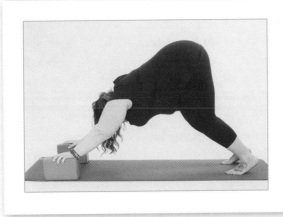

Amber Karnes:
Downward-Facing Dog Pose with Blocks

"With Downward-Facing Dog, putting blocks under my hands gives me more room to transition between poses in Sun Salutation because I have a larger body. I also bend my knees really deeply in Downward-Facing Dog to help my spine maintain length rather than trying to worry about getting my feet to the floor."

Wall Downward-Facing Dog Pose

From standing: This practice can also be done against a wall. Place your hands at shoulder height on the wall, hinge at your hips, and explore how far away to move your feet so that you can feel lengthening in your spine without being unsteady. Using a wall for Downward-Facing Dog Pose can allow you to experience the feeling of traction in your spine, opening in your arms and armpits, and strengthening your legs and feet without bringing your hands to the floor.

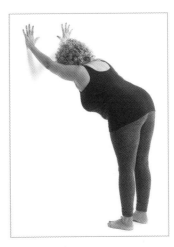

Upside-Down Dog Pose

From a bed or mat: If you're practicing in bed or on the mat and you don't want to put weight on your hands, feet, or knees, consider practicing an upside-down version of the pose. In this variation, try to recreate the energy of Downward-Facing Dog Pose. Instead of inverting your torso, you invert the lower half of your body. To come into the pose, sit on the floor with a bolster standing on end in front of you. Lean back onto one elbow and place your feet on top of the bolster. Lie back on the floor and raise your arms overhead. Can you still find the opening in your arms, length in your spine, and flexion in your hips? If you don't have a large bolster to prop under your legs, try placing your feet on the wall or the footboard of the bed.

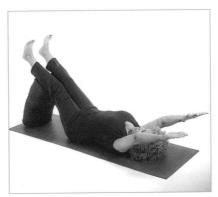

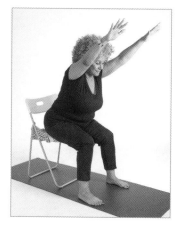

Chair Downward-Facing Dog Pose

From a chair: To experience Downward-Facing Dog Pose while sitting in a chair, begin by grounding your sit bones and feet in chair Mountain Pose. Raise your arms overhead as you inhale, and as you exhale hinge forward at the hips. From this strong foundation, see if you can bring in the energy of Downward-Facing Dog Pose by focusing on lengthening your spine and arms and incorporating hip flexion (hinging forward at the hips). The pose can also be done facing a wall. Bring your palms high up on the wall in front of you as you hinge forward. The wall can help to create the experience of traction in your spine and encourage the opening of your arms and armpit area.

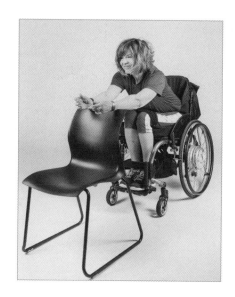

Mary Jo Fetterly:
Seated Downward-Facing Dog Pose with Support

"Downward-Facing Dog from a wheelchair with a chair in front allows me to get the full extension of the shoulder girdle, and the scapula can get pulled down at the same time. If I fall forward on my lap and try to do it without the chair, I go too far forward, so I lose that capacity to get at the shoulders and go into the lower back. So it's the perfect way to really release the shoulder girdle, the arm, the triceps some, and the biceps get worked, so it's all around good. Daily life needs to incorporate yoga if you're living in a chair, and that's one of the ways that you can do it."

SHOULDERSTAND (SARVANGASANA)

The main benefits of Shoulderstand, which can be explored with these variations, include:

- Resting the heart and lowering blood pressure
- Changing perspective
- Increasing venous blood flow and lymphatic return

Shoulderstand with Legs Up the Wall

From a mat: This pose has become synonymous with restorative yoga and is a welcome variation to Shoulderstand. Strictly speaking, raising your legs up the wall with your torso flat on the floor is not an inversion (except for the legs). But it can still rest your heart and increase venous blood flow and lymphatic return. Consider placing a bolster under the back of your pelvis to create a slight incline in your torso. Also, a blanket under your head can reduce the feeling of pressure there. To come into the pose, sit sideways to the wall with your left hip against the wall. Lower the right side of your body to the floor and scoot your buttock up to the wall. Roll onto your back and raise your legs up the wall. Hold for a few minutes if you're comfortable. You can also wrap your feet with a blanket to keep your legs together, your feet warm, and your heels cushioned against the wall.

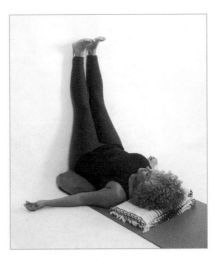

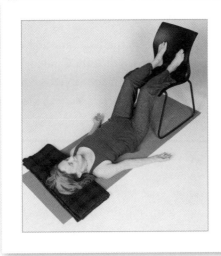

Linda Sparrowe: Shoulderstand with Legs on Chair

"I actually think this is one of the hardest poses to do, because it allows me to actually be in my body instead of doing something. Instead of do, do, do, it's a sense of just being. But the challenge is to allow my body to accept the gifts of gravity and allow me to come back into my back body so that my front brain isn't so active. So that is the key to this pose."

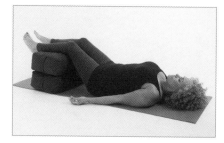

Shoulderstand with Legs Elevated

From a bed or mat: When practicing in a bed, your legs can be elevated on a pile of pillows or blankets so your feet are level with your knees. In a hospital bed, you can elevate them by raising the bottom portion of the bed. Some power wheelchairs offer this same opportunity, which is helpful for students who are practicing in their chairs.

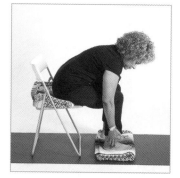

Seated Inversion

From a chair: When practicing yoga in a chair, it can be challenging to find a safe inversion. A Seated Forward Bend, in which you carefully hinge your torso forward at the hips and relax your head and neck, is one possibility. But that can be risky if you have osteoporosis in your neck. Blocks under your hands can help you feel more stable and prevent you from falling forward.

Raised Legs on Second Chair

From a chair: If you have enough flexibility in your legs, you can lean back in the chair and elevate your legs on a second chair that has a bolster on the seat. This will only invert your legs, but that can be soothing to your legs and feet if you sit a lot, and it can be relaxing for your entire system.

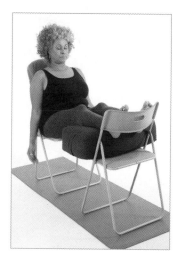

BRIDGE POSE (SETU BANDHA SARVANGASANA)

Bridge Pose is a gentle inversion that is actually a variation of Shoulderstand. It offers many of the same benefits without the challenge of supporting the weight of the body on the shoulders. In addition to creating a gentle inversion of the torso, Bridge Pose can help strengthen the legs, buttocks, and back.

Dynamic Bridge Pose

From a bed or mat: To make Bridge Pose more accessible, you can practice it dynamically. This means coming up and down with your breath. Bend your knees and plant your feet firmly on the mat. Inhale as you lift your hips toward the ceiling, and exhale as you slowly lower them back to the floor.

Repeat a few times with your breath. If it's comfortable, you can stay up in the pose for a few breaths. Make sure you're not straining your lower back and that you're engaging your legs. A block between your knees can help keep your legs aligned.

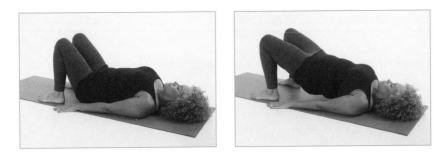

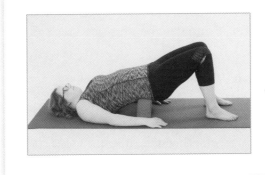

**Jessica Parsons:
Supported Bridge Pose**

"I like the Bridge Pose the most. It feels good. Sometimes with the block, it helps open my back. It helps open everything."

Low Shoulderstand

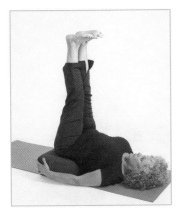

From a bed or mat: Come to Supported Bridge Pose with a bolster or block under your sacrum. Bend your knees toward your chest, then raise your legs toward the ceiling. This brings you into a low Shoulderstand, which offers many of the benefits of Shoulderstand without putting weight on your neck or stretching your neck too much. It also calls for core strength to hold your legs up in the air. If you're comfortable here, try to hold this pose for a minute or longer to increase the benefits.

CHILD'S POSE (BALASANA)

Child's Pose is a gentle inversion of the upper body as well as a forward bend. It offers an inward, quieting experience, but it can be uncomfortable and awkward for many people. Here are a few variations that can make it more accessible.

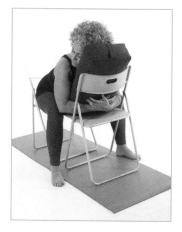

Chair Child's Pose While Hugging Bolster

From a chair: One option is a supported version of Child's Pose in a chair. For this practice, place a second chair in front of you with a bolster and folded blanket on it. Hinge forward at your hips and rest your chest on the bolster. You can rest your arms on the chair seat on either side of the bolster or hug the bolster. Use the blanket to elevate any portion of your chest or head that needs more space to make breathing easy and relaxed. You can rest your forehead on the bolster or turn your head to the side. If your head is to one side, turn it to the other side after a few breaths.

Chair Child's Pose

From a chair: Child's Pose can also be done in a chair by standing a bolster on end between your knees. Hinge forward with a long spine, and place your forearms on your thighs, holding the bolster in place with your hands. Try to rest your forehead on the end of the bolster. If it doesn't reach easily, place a block on top of the bolster. Making the connection between your head and the bolster can help to create that inward, restful feeling that inversions bring. Or you can place the bolster on your lap lengthwise with the block on top. In any of these variations, make sure your breath is relaxed the entire time.

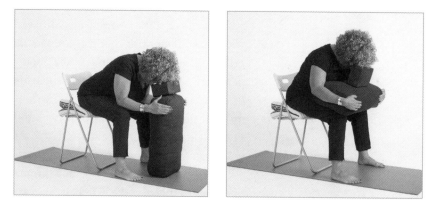

Child's Pose with Bolster

From a mat: When practicing Child's Pose, there are a few ways to adapt the practice that make it more comfortable and accessible. Try kneeling on a folded blanket with your toes off the end. This can help to avoid cramping in the feet because the toes are slightly lower than the ankles. You can place a folded blanket or bolster behind the backs of your thighs as well. Widen your knees so there's room for your belly when leaning forward. You can place a second bolster on the floor in front of you for support when you lean forward.

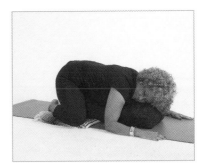

One of the most important parts of the practice is finding something to rest your forehead on. It can be a bolster, a block, the floor, or your forearms. The gentle pressure against your forehead can create the relaxing effect that is one of the hallmarks of inversions. Or turn your head to the side if that's more comfortable.

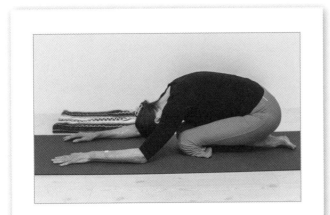

Marsha Danzig:
Accessible Child's Pose

"Child's Pose is both a resting pose and a challenge for me as an amputee. When I am taking or teaching a yoga class, I keep my prosthesis on. Since it does not bend deeply, I extend it behind me and do a 'half-Child's' with my other leg. At home, and when I teach amputees specifically, I often take off my prosthesis for Child's Pose. With the support of a folded blanket under my residual limb, I am able to fully surrender to the pose. That feels luxurious to me."

TWISTING 10

I HAD a series of lower back injuries culminating in a sprained sacroiliac (SI) joint that came from attempting to lift a student off the floor. As I healed from that injury, I found that twists were the most effective poses for releasing tension in that area in my body. Ironically, twists are considered potentially dangerous for the SI joint. This is an example of how hard it is to prescribe one type of pose or movement. I discovered there are ways to twist that are beneficial, just as there are ways to twist that can cause more harm.

Each of us is unique in our ability and in the way that an injury, disability, or illness manifests in our bodies. To address this, we need to be empowered with information as well as authority over our own bodies. For example, rather than following a set rule about how long to stay in a pose, you are encouraged to practice at your own pace and to stay in a pose for a length of time that feels good to you. When I teach public classes, I always encourage this inner listening. I often tell my students, "Listen to me, but don't listen to me."

The spine is the axis of our physical structure as well as the core of our nervous system. Sometimes these two essential aspects of the spine (supporting the physical structure of the body and protecting the nervous system) are at odds with each other.

As I mentioned, twists can also impact the junction of the spine and the pelvis, the SI joint, in a negative way. This joint needs to remain strong and stable and shouldn't be stretched. Unfortunately, many long-term yoga practitioners have problems with the SI joint, which may be related to continually practicing twisting poses and asymmetrical poses where the pelvis and spine are not moving as a unit. To address this issue, consider allowing your pelvis to move in twists, and try not to focus the force of twisting in your lower back. Let's consider some adapted twists that are more gentle on the SI joint.

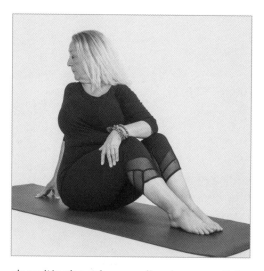

Camella Nair:
Seated Twist with Bent Knees

"I think this is a great pose because it gets me to actively sit in an upright position, and creates lots of inner body length. From that point I can decide whether the legs straighten, whether I do some crossing, whether I do binding, but essentially it's getting the SI joint in, inner body bright, and then working on the rotation from the thoracic spine.

It's not really about yoga poses. It's about becoming happier, and we're either consciously in the body or unconsciously in the body. It's not the stuff that we do for an hour and a half in a yoga class; it's about how we live, how we sit, how we walk, how we talk, all those things. So anything that we can do that's going to improve that is going to be good. And yoga isn't the only way, but it's a pretty cool way. It's a great methodology. It's karmic: there's a cause, and there's an effect. You do something positive that makes sense for your body, and things will improve. It's simple. It's not rocket science, is it really?"

HALF SPINAL TWIST (ARDHA MATSYENDRASANA)

A number of variations of this seated half spinal twist can make it more accessible. To assist with the starting position of sitting on the floor with the legs extended in front (Staff Pose [Dandasana]), you may benefit from sitting on a folded blanket or having a blanket under your knees. To avoid straining in the pose, it's important to use your arms only to support internal rotation rather than forcing it. Try to find a comfortable position where there is expansion in your chest, and your shoulders and chin are level.

It's important to continue to engage your breath to assist with the movement by focusing on lengthening your spine as you inhale and twisting as you exhale. If you have pronounced kyphosis (rounding in the upper back) or scoliosis (curve or twist in the spine), it's helpful to focus on lengthening rather than twisting. In this case, the practice can become a very subtle lifting and turning without much physical movement.

The position of the legs affects the amount of twist in the lower back and whether the SI joint is torqued. Here are some possible variations for the legs and lower body that can make this twist gentler. These instructions begin with twisting the torso to the right. Try to practice an equal amount of time on each side.

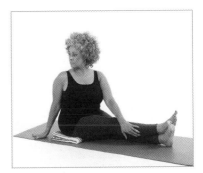

Spinal Twist with Ankles Crossed

From a mat: Sit in Staff Pose and keep both legs straight. Cross your right ankle over the left. Place your left hand on your right calf as you twist to the right.

Spinal Twist from a Cross-Legged Position

From a mat: Rather than beginning from Staff Pose, begin from a cross-legged position.

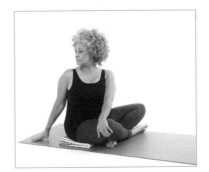

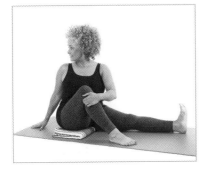

Spinal Twist with Uncrossed Legs

From a mat: Begin in Staff Pose, then open your legs wide apart. Bend your right knee and place your right foot on the floor. Keep your right foot in place and don't cross your legs as you twist.

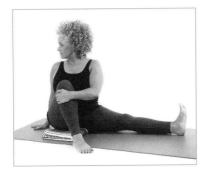

Spinal Twist Moving Hip

From a mat: To protect your SI joint, begin in Staff Pose and bend your right knee. Place your right foot on the floor without crossing your legs. Allow your right hip to move back an inch or so. Keeping your hip back, twist to the right, focusing on the twist in your middle and upper back and keep your lower back neutral.

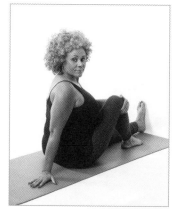

Spinal Twist Facing Wall

From a mat: Come into Staff Pose facing a wall with the soles of your feet against the wall. Keep your left foot against the wall during the pose. Bend your right knee and place your foot on the floor on either the right or left side of your left leg, depending on which is more comfortable for you.

Chair Twist with Legs Crossed

From a chair: To begin, come to chair Mountain Pose. To twist to the right, cross your right thigh over your left. Inhale, lengthen your spine, and begin to twist to the right, bringing your right hand to the back of the chair seat. Experience a gentle, even twist starting at your naval and rising up your spine through your neck to the top of your head. Don't force the twist with your arms. Instead, allow the deep core muscles to initiate the movement. Be sure to come out of the twist just as gently as you went into it, then practice on the other side.

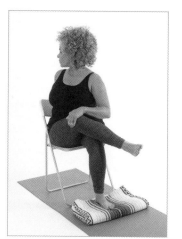

Chair Twist Sitting Sideways

From a chair: Alternatively, if your chair doesn't have arms, sit sideways with the back of the chair against your right arm. Cross your legs (but not if this is uncomfortable); inhale as you lengthen your spine, and exhale as you begin twisting to the right. Place your hands gently on the back of the chair to stabilize the twist without pulling yourself farther around with the strength of your arms. Take a few breaths and release. Repeat on the other side.

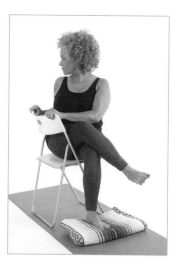

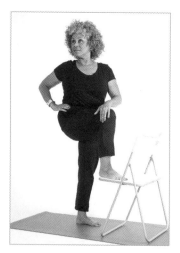

Standing Twist with Chair

From standing: Stand facing a chair in Mountain Pose. Make sure the chair is stable and, if possible, on a yoga mat for increased traction. Place your right foot on the seat of the chair and begin to twist to the right. Your right hand can be on your right hip and your left hand is on your right thigh. Inhale and lengthen your spine, and exhale and twist to the right. Look right with your eyes to gently twist your neck. Take a few breaths and then twist to the other side.

Standing Twist at Wall

From standing: A standing twist can be done using the wall instead of a chair. Stand sideways to the wall with your right shoulder touching it. Inhale and lengthen your spine, and exhale and twist to the right, placing your hands on the wall at shoulder height. To increase the stretch, cross your right leg over your left, and place your right foot on the other side of your left foot. Allow your spine and pelvis to move together so there's no strain on your SI joint. Take a few breaths and then repeat on the other side.

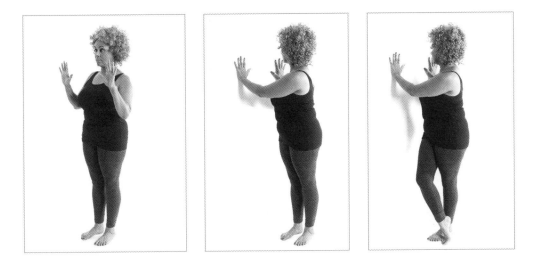

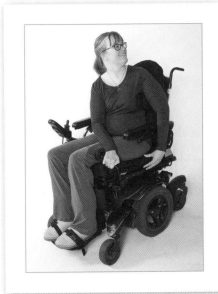

Jennifer Gasner: Chair Twist

"The twist allows me to create some space and movement in my spine, which feels really good since my spine remains basically static otherwise."

Revolved Abdomen Pose (Jathara Parivartanasana)

This pose is an effective way to get a twist to the middle back. It can also open the lower back and hips, as well as gently stretch the buttocks. Stretching these areas can be helpful for sciatica or piriformis syndrome (which is similar to sciatica but is caused by tightness in the piriformis muscle in the buttocks). Place a blanket between your legs to create alignment in your hips and slightly reduce the twist. The blanket also cushions your feet and ankles.

To protect your SI joint, be sure to move your pelvis and spine together. You can start by bending your knees, bringing your feet flat on the floor. Lift your hips and move them slightly to the left. Then lower your buttocks, bend your knees toward your chest, and lower your knees to the right. If your shoulders lift, place props under your legs until your shoulders are resting on the floor. Turn your head gently to the left. Repeat on the other side.

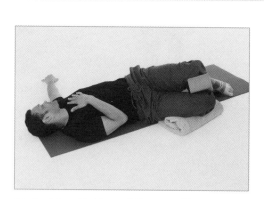

Miarco Tiama:
Lying Twist with Support

"I think that the lying twist has always worked for me and my body type, releasing lower back stress. Since I've had my back surgery, I still like to return to that posture, but there are days when it's just too tight, and I'm not able to bring my knee all the way down to the ground. When I take a bolster, this posture becomes completely accessible to me, and I'm able to then relax the inner groin and all the leg muscles that are worried about letting go. Then letting go, I can release that tension.

I'm able to dial in to where I need to be with my lower back and sacrum and not worry about being too loose or too tight. And then this release and letting go of all these worries, just because I can support my knee, allows me to do what I need to do. That's basically to breathe into my lower back and to release the lower vertebrae, which is the main goal of why I do this posture."

PART THREE

ACCESSIBLE
SUBTLE PRACTICES

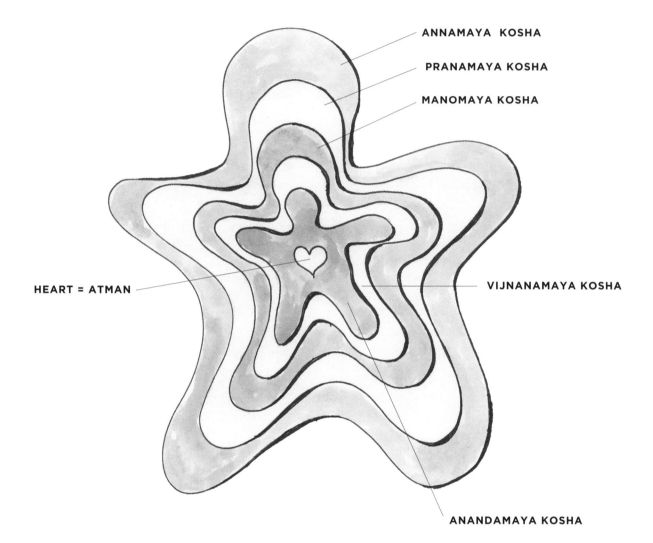

ANNAMAYA KOSHA

PRANAMAYA KOSHA

MANOMAYA KOSHA

VIJNANAMAYA KOSHA

HEART = ATMAN

ANANDAMAYA KOSHA

RELAXING 11

IN THE WEST, we talk about the mind-body connection, and scientific researchers are busy trying to prove that the mind has influence over the body. But isn't it common sense? Don't you feel it in your body when you're stressed or don't sleep well? Maybe it makes your muscles achy or gives you digestive problems. Does anxiety make your heart race or your breath shorten?

The connection between body and mind seems clear, and you can take advantage of this relationship in your yoga practice by working in both directions. You can work on the mind to affect the body, and you can work on the body to affect the mind.

In the yoga model of the human body, we are literally an expansion of energy moving at different levels of vibration. Like ice, water, and steam, which are all the same except the atoms are moving at different rates of vibration. You can compare the body to ice, the breath to water, and the mind to steam. There is really no difference between them, and what happens to one automatically affects the others. The subtle body is the most powerful level, expanding into the mind, the breath, and finally, the physical body. This model is the foundation on which all the yoga practices function.

We can work with these layers of being in a guided relaxation technique called yoga nidra, literally "yogic sleep." It's sometimes referred to as *Savasana* (Corpse Pose). Actually, *Savasana* is the physical posture, and yoga nidra is a guided meditation practice that you can do in that posture.

Yoga nidra is a progressive relaxation technique that is a journey through the layers of our being. There are five layers called *kosha* (sheaths or bodies), collectively known as *panca maya kosha*, which constitute our human embodiment. Like the layers of an onion or a Russian nesting doll, they expand from the astral body to the physical body.

From Outer to Inner: Pancamayakosha

The five kosha are:

1. *Annamaya kosha*, the physical body
2. *Pranamaya kosha*, the energy (breath) body
3. *Manomaya kosha*, the mental body
4. *Vijnanamaya kosha*, the wisdom body
5. *Anandamaya kosha*, the bliss body

To practice yoga nidra, you begin by tensing and releasing each part of your body. If you have a neurological disorder, like multiple sclerosis or Parkinson's disease, it may be helpful to focus on stretching and releasing each part, without tensing. Then mentally scan your body while keeping it still. Generally, move your awareness from your feet up and from outer to inner. Notice what happens when you bring your awareness to a part of your body. Can you feel more sensation and more energy there?

After scanning your body, notice your breath and then your mind. Finally, move into the stillness and experience the bliss body, the peace, anandamaya kosha, that is your essential nature. Spend a short time in silence before slowing coming out. Self-guided yoga nidra practice can be challenging, so you may want to download a recording of someone else leading it. Or you can even make your own recording of the practice exercise on page 132 and listen to it later. It can be very powerful to follow a meditation in your own voice.

Corpse Pose (Savasana)

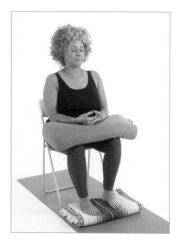

Corpse Pose can be surprisingly challenging because it can be hard to rest the busy mind. It helps if your body is supported with props. It also helps if your body is a comfortable temperature, the light is dim (or you can use an eye pillow), and you feel safe and secure. Covering yourself with a blanket, even when it's not very cold, can be effective. One of the most challenging parts of the practice is staying awake, but often falling asleep is exactly what the body needs. The only real issue with falling asleep is keeping track of the time or snoring if you're in a group class.

Chair Corpse Pose

From a chair: If Corpse Pose on a mat is not accessible to you, then you can practice yoga nidra while lying in bed or sitting in a chair. If you're practicing in a chair, make sure that you don't slip out if you fall asleep. To help with this, try moving your feet forward rather than having them directly under your knees. Or tie a yoga strap around your waist and the back of the chair like a seat belt. Some wheelchairs have built-in seat belts you can use. You can also place a blanket or bolster on your lap to rest your arms on. The added weight of the bolster can be soothing.

Chair Corpse Pose with Legs on Second Chair

From a chair: If it would be more comfortable, your feet can be raised on a bolster or on a second chair in front of you. Try placing a bolster or blanket behind your lower back, and lean back so you are gently reclining in the chair. Your arms can be resting in your lap or hanging down at your sides.

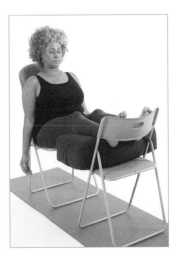

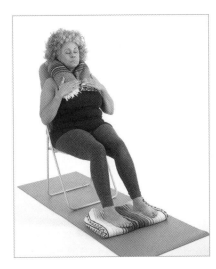

Chair Corpse Pose with Neck Support

From a chair: Check that your neck is well supported during the relaxation. You can roll a blanket and wrap it around your neck like a scarf to support your head like a neck pillow. Or use an airplane pillow to help support your head. You could also place your chair against a wall and have a blanket or pillow behind your head.

Corpse Pose on the Mat or Bed

From a bed or mat: If you're practicing on the floor or in bed, place a blanket or a small pillow under your head to try to keep your forehead and chin level, or your forehead slightly higher than your chin. You can also bend your knees and widen your feet with your knees leaning together. This can help lengthen your lower back if it's tender.

Another option is to place a bolster under your knees (or the backs of your thighs) to release your lower back. Experiment with the placement of the support under your legs to find a position where your

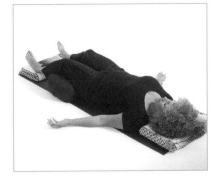

lower back is lengthened, and it creates a sensation of traction. You can add a rolled blanket under your heels or the backs of your wrists for added support.

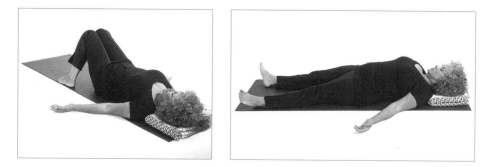

Inclined Corpse Pose

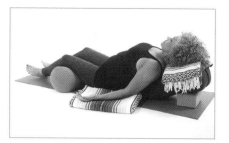

From a bed or mat: If you don't want to lie flat on the floor, you can lean back against a bolster propped at an angle with a block or two under the higher side. A blanket under your head and blankets under each arm provide additional support, as does a bolster under your knees. You can also practice while lying on your side if lying on your back is uncomfortable.

⁚⁚ *Try It: Guided Relaxation* ·

Find a comfortable position using one of the variations of Corpse Pose described here. You can cover your eyes with an eye pillow or darken the room. Cover yourself with a blanket if it's cold and if you enjoy the weight of the blanket on your body. You can record yourself reading the following directions or practice with another person. Once you learn it, you can guide yourself through it mentally.

- Begin by stretching out your right leg. Inhale, lift the leg just a little, and stretch it away from your body. Exhale and relax it back to the floor.
- Stretch out your left leg. Inhale, lift the leg just a little, and stretch it away from your body. Exhale and relax it back to the floor.
- Roll your legs from side to side and let them relax.
- Stretch out your right arm and spread your fingers wide. Inhale, lift the arm just a little, and stretch it away from your body. Exhale and relax it back to the floor.
- Stretch out your left arm and spread your fingers wide. Inhale, lift the

arm just a little, and stretch it away from your body. Exhale and relax it back to the floor.

- Roll your arms from side to side and let them relax.
- Inhale; tighten your buttocks. Exhale; let them relax.
- Inhale into your belly and your chest, allowing them to expand. Hold the breath for a moment, and let it go with a long sigh.
- Repeat.
- Squeeze your shoulders up toward your ears, and release.
- Press your shoulders down toward your feet, and release.
- Roll your head from side to side, and let it relax back to center.
- Inhale and squeeze your face, making it small.
- Exhale and stretch your eyes and mouth wide open.
- Repeat.
- Move your jaw from side to side, open and close your mouth.
- Relax your face and your entire body.
- Bring your awareness down to your feet, and notice sensation there.
- Slowly move your awareness up into your lower legs, knees, and thighs.
- Awareness into your buttocks, hips, and pelvis.
- Awareness into your abdomen and chest, noticing sensation there.
- Awareness into your hands and fingers, forearms, upper arms, and shoulders.
- Awareness into the back of your body, where it is being supported on the floor, bed, or chair.
- Awareness to your lower back, middle back, and upper back.
- Awareness to your neck, throat, and jaw.
- Bring your awareness into your face—jaw, tongue, cheeks, nose, eyes, eyebrows, and forehead.
- Awareness to the sides of your head and ears, the back of your head, and the top of your head.
- Become aware of your entire body.
- Notice your breath.
- Notice thoughts and emotions in your mind.
- Become aware of the witness itself.
- (Spend a few minutes in silence if you're comfortable.)
- To come out, bring your awareness back to your breath.
- Stretch out your limbs, and either roll to the side and rest, or sit up slowly.
- Take a moment to notice how you feel.

BREATHING 12

USUALLY, *pranayama* is translated into English as "breathing practices," but that translation doesn't quite do it justice. Pranayama is better understood as expansion of *prana*, which is the Sanskrit word for "energy" or "life force." In a sense, pranayama is similar to acupuncture, which is also concerned with the movement of energy (*qi*). You could even compare the use of needles in acupuncture with the use of the breath in pranayama. The breath is the tool that we use to work with the life force within us. With this in mind, you can approach pranayama with a subtler awareness—not only are you working with the breath, but with life force itself.

According to the Yoga Sutras of Patanjali, as the result of practicing pranayama, "the veil over the inner light is destroyed" (2.52).[1] Pranayama has the capacity to remove this veil, which is made up of all the busy thoughts in the mind. This is because the breath and the mind move together, so when you slow your breath, you slow your mind. In this way pranayama prepares you for the deep concentrated awareness of meditation. Instinctively, we know the breath is a tool for working with the mind. If someone is upset or emotional, the first thing we do is tell them to take a deep breath.

Ironically, pranayama is often left out of public yoga classes. It may be because these practices are subtle and call for a level of patience that can make them seem advanced. But the opposite is true; these practices are accessible to all of us if we understand them. Ideally, after practicing some asana to get the energy moving in your body, you can practice *savasana* (or guided relaxation) and then come to a seated position on the floor or in a chair for pranayama and meditation. Or you can practice them in bed.

Sometimes stored emotions and memories are released during pranayama because of the relationship between breath and mind. So be sure to practice gently and slowly. Also, notice if you want to avoid practicing or feel like it's boring. Sometimes, feeling bored is the mind's way of avoiding something it doesn't want to look at. And that's okay. Don't force anything in pranayama, and if painful emotions or memories surface, stop practicing and reach out for support.

Also, if you feel lightheaded, dizzy, or anxious from pranayama, you should stop and return your breath to normal. If you have chronic obstructive pulmonary disease (COPD), other lung diseases, or anxiety, you need to approach these practices with care, making sure that you're not straining at any time. In these situations, working with a yoga teacher in person may be a safer approach.

A steady, comfortable posture is important during both pranayama and meditation, so that you can turn your awareness within and experience subtle shifts happening. Unless you're using your hands as part of the breathing practice, they can be resting on your knees or in your lap. Or if you prefer, you can touch your index fingers to your thumbs to create chin mudra. Mudras can help keep the mind focused by bringing awareness to the subtle ways that energy moves in the body. Here are some possible seated postures for pranayama and meditation.

SEATED

Cross-Legged with Rolled Blanket

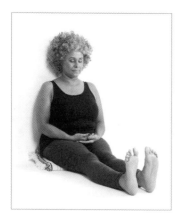

From a mat: You can sit cross-legged on a cushion on the floor, with a rolled blanket between your knees and ankles. This provides support for your hips and also protects your ankles. Focus on lengthening your spine and moving your shoulders back and away from your ears. Try to keep your chin level with the floor and relax your face. Feel your spine lengthening as you inhale, and try to relax the rest of your body as you exhale.

Cross-Legged with Blocks

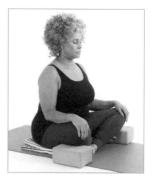

From a mat: As you are sitting cross-legged, you can also use blocks under your knees and angle them in whatever way is most comfortable.

Back to Wall

From a mat: You can sit back against a wall with your legs extended in front of you.

Thunderbolt Pose (Vajrasana)

From a mat: Straddle a bolster and sit back toward your heels in Thunderbolt Pose. To reduce the risk of cramping in your feet, it can be helpful to have a blanket under your legs with your toes coming off the edge of the blanket.

Chair Mountain Pose

From a chair: Sit in chair Mountain Pose with a blanket or bolster on your lap. Rest your hands on the bolster or blanket.

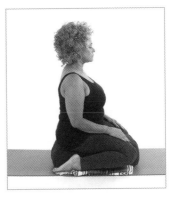

Diaphragmatic Breathing (Deergha Swasam)

To build a foundation in pranayama, it is helpful to begin by learning to breathe more deeply and efficiently. This is referred to as diaphragmatic breathing, or yogic breathing. It's important to use the diaphragm to its full potential, since it's the main breathing muscle in the body. Otherwise you're mostly using the auxiliary breathing muscles of your chest and neck, which is referred to as chest breathing, or reverse breathing.

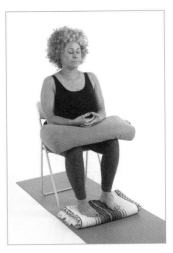

The diaphragm is a large muscle that separates the chest cavity from the abdominal cavity. Its movement is essential for breathing, and the rhythmic flow of the diaphragm benefits many other systems of the body. As the diaphragm moves, it encourages venous blood flow, massages the abdominal organs, and helps to pump lymph (the fluid of the immune system). It creates a flowing rhythm within the body, like waves breaking on a beach and receding back into the ocean.

Diaphragmatic breathing can be practiced with one hand on your belly to feel the movement there as you breathe in and out. On the inhalation, the diaphragm contracts and presses down on the top of the abdominal organs. In response, the abdominal organs move forward, which is why you feel your belly moving forward. On the exhalation, the diaphragm relaxes, which allows your belly to move back in toward your spine. It's helpful to remember that the breath moves with the diaphragm in this way: inhale, diaphragm contracts; exhale, diaphragm relaxes.

Pay special attention to lengthening the exhalation, because this will allow for the complete relaxation of your diaphragm. It also allows for maximum air exchange by creating space for fresh air to come in during the next inhalation. This extended exhalation can create a sense of release and relaxation in your entire body and has a variety of other health benefits. This is because deep, rhythmic breathing stimulates the vagus nerve, which is part of the parasympathetic nervous system and tells the whole body to relax. The following practices focus on increasing breath awareness and deepening the breath. Start slowly and with care, remembering that the goal is to expand energy. This happens through subtle shifts rather than big changes, and it requires practice and gentleness.

Weighted Breathing

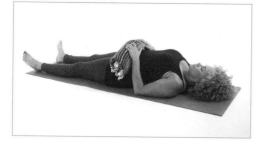

From a bed or mat: You can practice deep breathing while lying in Corpse Pose with a folded blanket or bolster on your abdomen. Use the weight of the prop on your abdomen to connect with the movement of your diaphragm. Feel the prop move up on each inhalation and down on each exhalation as the movement of your diaphragm is transferred to your abdominal organs.

Inclined Corpse Pose

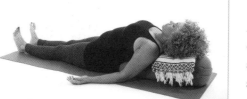

From a bed or mat: To expand your chest, you can practice diaphragmatic breathing in an inclined Corpse Pose. Place a bolster under the back of your ribcage, in line with your spine, and a blanket under your head. A block under the top of the bolster will create a gentle incline to support your back. Allow the bolster to expand the front of your chest and create space for deeper breathing.

Crocodile Pose (Makarasana)

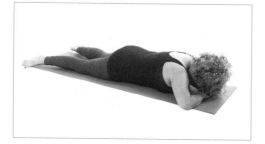

From a mat: Lie on your abdomen in Crocodile Pose. Cross your hands under your head with your cheek to the side. You can point your toes outward or however is most comfortable for you. Connect with the feeling of your abdomen against the floor. Notice how your abdomen presses into the floor during the inhalation, as it moves forward. On the exhalation, feel your abdomen moving away from the floor.

Holding Chest and Belly

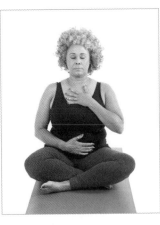

From a chair, bed, or mat: To deepen the breath, you can expand it in three sections: abdomen, chest, and collarbones. Place one hand on your belly and the other hand on your chest just under your collarbones. Exhale first. Then inhale and feel the breath moving your abdomen forward. Then feel the breath rising into your chest and all the way to the top of your lungs. On the exhalation, feel the breath leaving your chest and slowly emptying from your abdomen. Repeat a few times and feel the breath filling your lungs from the bottom up and releasing from the top down.

Or simply notice whatever movement your lungs naturally make. But try to deepen the breath so that you feel all three areas of your lungs filling and emptying. Eventually, these three parts blend into one long, deep breath.

Hands on Ribcage

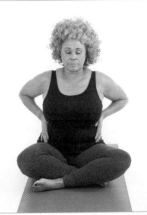

From a chair, bed, or mat: To experience the fullness of the breath, try placing your hands on your rib cage. Either move your elbows out to the sides and bring your hands to your side ribs, or give yourself a hug under your chest and hold on to your ribs. Exhale, then inhale and feel your rib cage expanding in all directions. Focus on the expanding sideways and backward. This opening in the ribcage allows the diaphragm muscle to expand outward as it flattens.

Hands on Head

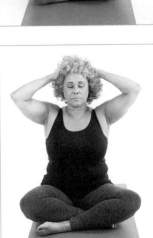

From a chair, bed, or mat: You can also try placing your hands on your head with your shoulders relaxed. Hold your head gently but firmly, connecting to the bones of the skull. Exhale, and then as you inhale, see if you notice a slight expansion of your skull. On the exhalation, try to feel your skull gently contract. Take a few breaths, connecting to the expansion and contraction in your skull and in your whole body as you breathe.

One way to deepen the exhalation in diaphragmatic breathing is to practice inhaling once and exhaling twice. It's important to do this practice in a relaxed way, without straining.

- Sit comfortably and become aware of the breath.
- Take a comfortable inhalation.
- Exhale slowly, pause.
- Now see if you can exhale gently again, releasing just a little more air.
- Inhale slowly and deeply.
- Repeat a few times.
- Then relax the breath and notice how you feel.

· ⁑

OCEAN BREATHING (UJJAYI)

To lengthen the breath, it's helpful to learn how to control the breath in your throat. This practice is called ocean breathing and is essential for progressing in pranayama. To better understand this technique, you can pretend to fog up a mirror in front of you by making a long "hhaa" sound with your mouth open. Then close your mouth and try to make that same sound. This light wheezing sound is the result of air passing through the reduced opening in your throat.

By reducing the size of the opening, the air takes longer to enter and exit your lungs. The result is that the breath is longer and slower. The sound produced can be compared to the sound of the wind or the ocean, and those images can be used to help inspire you to practice.

It can be helpful to begin using ocean breathing on the exhalation, since that's the part of the breath we're focusing on lengthening in pranayama. Feel the breath moving into your lungs on the inhalation from the bottom up, like a wave rising up on the beach; on the exhalation, use ocean breathing as the breath recedes from the top down, like a wave returning to the ocean.

Alternate Nostril Breathing (Nadi Suddhi)

Alternate nostril breathing is known by a few different Sanskrit names, including *nadi suddhi,* Anuloma Viloma and Sukha Purvaka. According to yogic subtle anatomy, this practice balances energy in the body, particularly in the right and left hemispheres of the brain. Each nostril is correlated with the opposite hemisphere of the brain, and this energetic balance is experienced as peacefulness in the mind. Scientists are studying the impact of alternate nostril breathing on the brain, and although it's unclear how it works, the practice definitely has a calming effect on the nervous system.[2]

From a chair, bed, or mat: Check your posture, and try to make your neck and spine long before beginning this practice. To begin alternate nostril breathing, make a gentle fist with your right hand and extend the last two fingers and thumb. Or you can use your left hand or a different finger combination, such as the index finger and thumb. Bring your hand to your nose, close your right nostril, and exhale from the left nostril. Inhale from the left, switch nostrils, and exhale from the right. Continue with this pattern of exhale-inhale-switch, breathing gently and slowly.

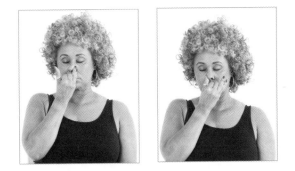

Once the pattern is comfortable, you can lengthen the exhalation using ocean breathing. Eventually try to make the exhalation twice as long as the inhalation. Be sure there is no straining or shortness of breath. If there is, return the breath to normal. Practice for a few minutes and then release your hand, relax the breath, and notice how you feel.

Alternatively, if using your hand is not possible, the practice can be done just using the mind. Imagine the breath moving in this same pattern, out and in from one nostril at a time. This is actually a more advanced form of the practice because it takes mental concentration to experience the subtle movement of the breath and to stay focused. It's a very helpful technique if you want to practice in public, like on a bus or a plane. After practicing alternate nostril breathing, or any pranayama, it is useful to take a moment and notice how your mind and body are feeling before moving on to the next practice. I encourage you to explore different accessible pranayama techniques, which can give you access to the peace of mind that is at the core of yoga practice and are a powerful antidote to the stress of everyday life.

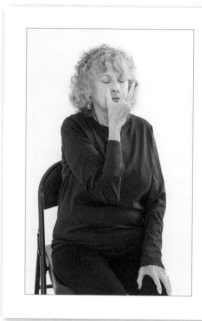

**Kalyani Baral:
Alternate Nostril Breathing
with Index Finger and Thumb**

"Yoga has given me an inner spiritual life for forty-five years that I never even imagined. The practices of Integral Yoga—including asanas, deep relaxation, breathing techniques, and most importantly, meditation—has assisted me in coping with many health issues over my seventy years."

MEDITATING 13

THE YOGA TEACHINGS often talk about controlling the mind, but anyone who's ever tried to meditate knows that trying to control the mind is like trying to stop a train that's going eighty miles an hour. After thirty years of trying to meditate, I'm done fighting with myself. I barely try to stop my mind anymore when I'm meditating because it feels like an uphill battle. Instead, I'm trying to make peace with my mind by learning to have a healthy relationship with the person I'm always with—myself.

I've started a new meditation technique that goes against everything I've been taught (don't tell anyone). I say, "Yes!" to my thoughts, rather than a constant "No." This technique comes from my experience raising kids; at least, it worked when they were younger. Now that they're teenagers, it's a little more complicated.

Back then, if they were doing something I didn't want them to do, like drawing on the wall, I'd redirect them. I might say, "I see you're wanting to draw. How about drawing on this nice paper instead?" rather than yelling at them, "Stop drawing on the wall!" In fact, I found that if there was a lot of energy behind my yelling, "Stop," they would get more excited about misbehaving, and sometimes that behavior would continue even longer. A warm redirect was the most potent way to encourage positive behavior with my kids and also with my own mind.

What I've noticed in meditation is that my mind is usually telling a story, so I try to listen. Doesn't everyone want to be listened to, to be heard? I try to offer that loving presence to my own mind, just like I would actively listen to someone I love. When I'm actively listening, I pay close attention to what's being said as well as the energy behind the words. In active listening, it's also important to avoid reacting and thinking about my response. Instead, I listen to myself. I try to simply remain present with whatever is going on in my thoughts, in my body, and in my heart: listening, feeling, being present.

The other thing that no one tells you about meditation is that you may actually have a lot of great ideas. That's because in meditation, if the mind calms down a little, the voice of your heart may rise up with the creativity that is at the core of your being. I love to listen to those thoughts, and I don't tell them to go away.

I want my meditation to be a time for inner peace but also an expansion of my heart, which may speak to me in words or in feelings. Creativity and spirituality are really the same thing. In both, we are allowing the energy of creation to move through us. We just need to learn how to get out of our own way.

⠢ *Try It: Making Friends with the Mind Meditation* . . . .

Check your posture and prepare for a short meditation in whatever fashion is most comfortable for you. This could mean lighting a candle or sitting in a special spot.

- Deepen the breath just a little.
- Notice how your body feels by doing a quick body scan.
- Notice what kind of energy is in your body.
- Do you feel nervous, relaxed, tired, or something else?
- Notice if there are any emotions and allow yourself to experience them.
- If an emotion arises, say the word *yes*.
- Notice if there are any thoughts in the mind.
- If a thought arises, say the word *yes*.
- Whenever you notice an emotion or thought, say the word *yes*.
- Spend a few minutes practicing this technique.
- To finish, notice how you feel.
- Take a few full breaths and thank yourself for spending this time practicing meditation.

. . . . ⠢

YOGA MEDITATION

It's interesting that today, yoga and meditation are considered two distinct practices. Throughout the history of yoga, up until just a few decades ago, a discussion of yoga would automatically include meditation as the ultimate practice. This is because yoga practice is defined as the effort to steady the mind, as noted in the Yoga Sutras (1:13).[1] But over the past few decades, Western yoga practitioners have shifted more of the focus to asana and physical practice.

Sutra 2.29 states that Ashtanga Yoga, the eight limbs of yoga, are:

1. *Yama* (abstinence)
2. *Niyama* (observance)
3. *Asana* (posture)
4. *Pranayama* (breath control)
5. *Pratyahara* (sense withdrawal)
6. *Dharana* (concentration)
7. *Dhyana* (meditation)
8. *Samadhi* (contemplation, absorption, or super-conscious states) [2]

It can be helpful to consider the role that meditation plays in classical yoga. In Patanjali's Yoga Sutras, one of the most well-known teachings is called "Ashtanga Yoga," or the Eight Limbs of Yoga (2:29). Patanjali offers a clear path toward enlightenment in this description of practice that moves from external, outwardly focused practices to more internal, reflective ones.

He begins with the ten precepts of yama and niyama, which offer clarity about how to live as a yogi in the world so that you can keep your peace in all situations—starting with nonviolence, truthfulness, and not stealing. These teachings can be understood as both inner and outer ethical practices. For example, by not causing harm, you keep your mind peaceful. By not lying, you prevent a lot of worry and overthinking that would be needed to keep a lie going. By living in an ethical way, you can also offer service to the world by not adding to the pain and suffering that already exists. For example, veganism reduces harm to animals and reduces global warming.

Patanjali continues with the third limb, asana or posture, and the fourth, pranayama or breathing practice. Next is sense withdrawal (pratyahara), an essential first step in meditation. Ask yourself, what's the first thing you do when you go to meditate? Do you dim the lights, put down your phone, sit down and close your eyes? All of these preparatory steps are designed to reduce sensory stimulation. You can think of pratyahara as thought prevention. Face it, it's really hard to meditate while scrolling through Facebook.

Next, Patanjali offers the sixth limb of Ashtanga Yoga: concentration (dharana). He describes dharana as "the binding of the mind to one place, object or idea" (3:1).[3] It's interesting that Patanjali offers so many options to focus on here, as if to show us that his interest is in the technique itself, not necessarily the object we choose to focus on. This open-minded approach is what makes the yoga practices so inclusive to people from all faith traditions. You could even say this is why yoga is not a religion, but rather a spiritual practice where everyone is welcome.

Some common objects for meditation are the breath, Sanskrit mantras, body sensations, a location in the body such as the heart or third eye, a candle flame, mandalas, images of deities, or a concept such as love or peace. Concentration means trying to focus the mind on that object. Although it sounds simple, it's actually extremely challenging, and as I mentioned, I've stopped forcing my mind to comply. Rather, I work with my mind to learn how to rest on the object of meditation.

It's like a dog that runs around and plays frantically but eventually likes to rest in its own dog bed. Or even better, you can think of the devotion a dog has for you (if you're a dog person), and how your dog follows you around with complete dedication. The mind is like the dog—dedicated to the object of concentration. So choosing an object that you love for meditation is the key to successful concentration. This way the practice becomes relaxing and enjoyable rather than a chore.

The seventh limb is meditation (dhyana), or being in the flow. This is the experience of timelessness, where the mind is completely absorbed in an activity. It's an experience that happens for all of us naturally throughout the day. Can you think of particular activities that cultivate that experience of dropping into the moment and being in the flow?

Often, creative activities such as art, music, and dance help to bring the mind into the moment. Interestingly, dangerous sports, like rock-climbing, surfing, and skiing, can also cultivate this experience by forcing the mind to be present—since otherwise you may get hurt! While these activities may not always create the experience of being in the flow, yoga is specifically designed for this purpose. All that we do in the name of yoga helps to bring the mind to a single-pointed focus.

Eventually, that focus flows naturally into enlightenment (samadhi), or so I'm told. The eighth limb of yoga is a state of self-realization, of connecting with the essence of who we are rather than continually identifying with the thoughts in the mind. Ironically, samadhi is really more about stopping our identification, or union, with thoughts rather than creating union with the true self. The true self is who we are. It's already there, listening and watching as the silent witness. To experience the true self, we give the mind something to focus on so it becomes calm, and then the spirit can shine through like the sun shining through the clouds of the mind.

Meditation Practices

Once I make the time for meditation, I usually find a great feeling of relief, like a weight lifted off my shoulders. But that's not always the case. There are times when meditation simply brings up whatever emotion I'm struggling with or trying to avoid. So when I'm going through a difficult time, it can be even harder to make myself sit for meditation.

Giving myself the power to choose when and how I want to practice is key to my sense of empowerment and, ultimately, my increased self-awareness. Meditation can feel overwhelming if it brings up stored trauma or anxiety. In that case, it may be helpful to focus on more active practices like asana and breathing and to only incorporate short periods of silence. When beginning a meditation practice, it's important to use common sense and be kind to yourself. Actually, it's always important to use common sense and be kind to yourself, and spiritual practice is no exception.

There are many ways to approach the mind, and it's helpful to explore different techniques and discover which practice feels most comfortable and accessible for you. For example, if you don't feel comfortable with a Sanskrit mantra, a neutral practice, like meditation on the breath, might be more effective. Or explore your own spiritual beliefs and traditions to find a practice that works for you.

It's also important to find a comfortable position for meditation. Generally, it's helpful to sit upright, either on the floor or in a chair. But resting in Corpse Pose is fine as long as you can stay awake. You can review the different options for seated positions in chapters 3 and 12.

Breath Meditation

The most universal focus for meditation is the breath itself, since it is always in the present moment. By focusing on the breath, the mind is brought back into the present, which is the only time when we can actually feel happiness and peace. When focusing on the breath, the mind can observe the physical sensations of breathing, focus on the energetic experience of the breath moving up and down the spine, or focus on the feeling of the whole body expanding on the inhalation and contracting on the exhalation.

❖ Try It: Breath Meditation

- Sit in a comfortable position with a long spine. Relax your body. Close your eyes or just relax them.
- Bring your awareness to the breath coming in through your nose on the inhalation.
- Feel the air, slightly cool, moving through your sinuses, down your throat, and expanding your lungs.

- On the exhalation, notice the air leaving your lungs through the airways, slightly warmer now at the nostrils.
- Spend a few minutes observing all the sensations of breathing. What muscles are moving? What do you feel in your body?
- If your mind wanders, notice that and come back gently to your breath.
- Open your eyes and notice how you feel.

⋮⋮

Mantra Meditation

Mantras are sound vibrations designed to focus the mind. All Sanskrit mantras are considered to be aspects of the universal hum OM. If you have a devotional nature, you can explore the relationships between different Hindu deities and their related mantras. Or you can focus on a universal mantra such as OM SHANTI, HARI OM, or SO HUM.

When using a mantra, it's helpful to feel a keen interest in the sound or the meaning of the sound. This interest will help bring the mind to rest on the mantra, and over time it may begin to repeat the mantra automatically. Each time the mind wanders off to another thought, gently bring it back to the mantra without criticism or frustration. This gentle but consistent training will allow the mind to get quieter and quieter. It can be very helpful to coordinate the mantra with the breath in whatever pattern feels comfortable for you. You can experiment with the mantra SO HUM, which means "I am That," and is also simply the sound of the breath.

⋮⋮ Try It: SO HUM Meditation

- Sit comfortably and relax your body. Close your eyes or soften your gaze.
- Become aware of your breath.
- Inhale, and mentally repeat the sound "so."
- Exhale, and mentally repeat the sound "hum."
- Continue with this practice for a few minutes.
- As you practice, try to listen to your breath making the sound "so hum."
- After a few minutes, take a deep inhalation, and exhale slowly, opening or refocusing your eyes.
- Notice how you feel.

⋮⋮

Visual Meditation

Visual meditation can be effective if you are a very visual person or in combination with the other techniques I've already described. For this type of meditation, you can use a candle flame, flower, picture of a deity, or mandala. Try focusing your eyes on the object for a little while, and then close your eyes and picture the object in your mind.

⁙ *Try It: Light Meditation*

- Sit comfortably in front of a candle flame at eye level.
- Check your posture and relax your breath.
- Stare at the flame for about a minute. (Blink as needed.)
- Feel that the light is filling you with peace and warmth.
- Close your eyes and notice the image of the flame on your retina.
- Continue to feel the light expanding within.
- Bring in awareness of your breath or a mantra.
- Open or close your eyes as you like.
- After a few minutes, close your eyes.
- Rub your palms together briskly.
- Palm your eyes with your warm hands.
- Release and open your eyes.
- Notice how you feel.

One other useful technique in meditation is to focus on a point inside the body, such as the heart or third-eye center. This is helpful in combination with breath or mantra meditation. Although we're trying to focus the mind, it can be helpful to engage the mind fully with a combination of practices that work together. For example, synchronizing the breath and mantra, as well as bringing awareness to the heart or third eye.

I encourage you to experiment with different techniques, different times of day, and different seated positions. Eventually, try to settle on a relatively consistent practice. For example, sitting in the same place, at the same time of day, for the same length of time. A great way to begin is to add 5 minutes of meditation after you do some asanas and breathing practices.

Try to make meditation a special time for yourself. Do you value yourself enough to spend time with yourself? Notice when your mind resists, what it chooses to do instead of meditating. Or are you valuing your family members, your work, or even your Facebook friends more than your own self? Can you use meditation to give yourself the love and care that you give to others?

PART FOUR

ACCESSIBLE YOGA PRACTICE

BUILDING A HOME PRACTICE 14

THE MOST CHALLENGING thing about creating a personal yoga practice is setting aside time for yourself. I remember that when my kids were younger, I would look longingly at adults who didn't have kids and imagine the days when I could do whatever I wanted, whenever I wanted. Between kids and work there was barely a moment left for me. With young children you can't even go to the bathroom in peace! But even one moment of awareness can be turned into a pause button for self-care and reconnection. One moment of focusing on the breath or exploring sensation in the body.

The truth is, I'm really no use to anyone if I don't take care of myself. I can push and push, but in the end I end up burned out or sick. Personally, I struggle with lower back issues and occasional anxiety. These both flare up when I don't invest time in self-care, and the main part of my self-care is yoga and meditation.

When my kids were young, I struggled to find time to practice. Usually it was when they were napping. Sometimes that meant not showering, but it was worth it. When I try to take care of others all day without taking care of myself, it just wears me down. I have no energy left for anyone or anything.

Even with a short regular yoga practice, you may begin to feel some benefit, but the key is the regularity of practice. Going to an hour-and-a-half-long yoga class every few weeks is great, and I highly recommend it, but the most benefit comes from bringing yoga into your life as a part of your daily routine. Any time of day is fine, but traditionally the beginning or end of the day are considered most conducive for practice—in particular, sunrise and sunset. If possible, I suggest starting with 15 minutes a day, first thing in the morning, before you eat breakfast or at the end of the day before dinner. (It's generally better not to practice right after you eat.)

One approach I recommend for building a home practice is what I call the "5/5/5 method." This is where you practice 5 minutes of asana, 5 minutes of conscious breathing, and 5 minutes of relaxation or meditation every day. This surprises a lot of people who think that to do yoga you need to have a lot of time and do lots of poses. I find that the subtle practices can often bring more immediate benefit and therefore will encourage regular practice. Over time you can extend the asana portion, but try to stick with at least 5 minutes of breathing and 5 minutes of relaxation or meditation each day.

Another challenge for creating a home yoga practice is finding a physical space in which to do it. If you don't have a space that you can dedicate to yoga, then you need to be a little more creative. You can practice in a chair, in bed, or on a small space on the floor. What's most important is that you find a space where you can truly relax and not be disturbed for the time you're practicing. Accessible Yoga is about making the most out of what you have: your time and energy, as well as your space and resources.

If possible, choose one location where you can practice regularly and allow this to become a sacred space for you. If you feel inspired to create an altar, that can be a useful practice in itself. An altar is like a spiritual mirror. It is a reflection of the essence within us, the higher consciousness. An altar can simply be the corner of a desk or a window sill. You can add pictures of people who inspire you, rocks, shells, anything that makes you happy. If you like, you can have a candle or some flowers.

The main thing is to create a space that is supportive of relaxation. After a while the space can even support you. If you practice in one place for a period of time, that place will begin to remind you of your practice. When you aren't feeling well, or if you're anxious, you can go into that space, and it will remind you of how relaxed you felt previously. Building a sacred space like this can become a preventive measure for reducing future stress.

Accessible Props

The power of yoga lies in the ability to turn within and connect with yourself. This can only occur when the body feels safe, and props are the way to bring in that feeling of safety and support. It's not hard to imagine how pushing the body beyond its natural limitations or feeling competitive can put you in an unsafe situation. So using props can actually make your practice more advanced.

Unfortunately, yoga props can be expensive, but there are many things around your house you can use if you don't have access to traditional yoga props. In fact, my favorite yoga prop is a wall—and those are pretty easy to find! I also love using yoga blankets to support my body, but you don't have to have a special yoga blanket. Look for any blanket that is on the firm side in cotton or wool, or you can use a large towel. Also, a regular bed pillow works well if you don't have blankets or yoga bolsters.

Remember, there are other props that you may not even realize you already have, like a chair, a bed, even the floor or the doorway. Here's a list of some everyday items you can use in place of yoga props:

ELEMENTS OF A YOGA PRACTICE

There are two main components to a yoga practice: the physical poses (asana) and the subtler practices of relaxation, breathing, and meditation. These two parts of practice—the physically active and the mentally calming—form a kind of yin/yang of yoga. In fact, another word for yoga is *balance*. Yoga is about effort and release. In your practice, it's helpful to find a balanced approach. Do some active poses and then some relaxation. Let's consider these two areas for a moment and figure out how to come up with an enjoyable home practice that will offer you a respite during your day and give you energy for what's to come.

Often, my asana practice is all warm-ups, and that's okay. Remember, there aren't any yoga police watching to make sure you do traditional poses in their "full expression," especially if you're practicing at home. Instead, you can begin to explore what practices will help you find balance in your body and in your mind. The elements of a practice are:

1. Centering
2. Movement (warm-ups and asanas)
3. Relaxation, breathing, meditation

In yoga more isn't always better. There is power in subtlety, and in fact, the more subtle the practice is, the more powerful it is. A good example of this is pranayama (breathing practices), where the ultimate goal is slowing the breath and finding still points between the breaths. In those quiet moments, the breath reflects a calm and peaceful mind, which is what we're really working toward. So you could even say that the goal of the breathing practices is to stop breathing! It sounds funny, but it's true. Subtle is stronger. Stillness is advanced.

The focus of yoga practice is cultivating an experience of alert relaxation, or relaxed alertness. This may be a new experience, because usually we overly

---

If you don't have . . .

- *A yoga mat*, try practicing directly on a clean wood floor with a towel under your head. Or on a carpet if it's not too slippery.

- *A yoga bolster*, try rolling a bed pillow into a cylinder and tying it with a belt.

- *A yoga block*, try a stack of books or a low stool. Or use the seat of a chair or the wall for support.

- *A yoga strap*, try a belt, scarf, or tie. Even a sock will work.

- *A yoga blanket*, try using a bed pillow or folded towel.

caffeinate ourselves to get through the day and then come home at night and crash. Personally, I know that my days often feel like energetic roller coaster rides, up and down, and I'm constantly trying to make my internal experience match the activity I'm engaged in. Sometimes that means going to teach a yoga class when I'm feeling tired or lying in bed at night and trying to fall asleep when my mind is wide awake. Yoga can help us balance our energy by finding a neutral ground where we are energized but peaceful.

The challenge with asana practice is to build strength and energy without injury. This can only come through the development of internal awareness (interoception), so you become sensitive to what you need in that moment, so you become intimate with yourself. Practicing asana based on external goals is much less effective; for example, the intention "I want to look like that model on the cover of the yoga magazine" wouldn't help as much as "I'm going to use this time to experience what's happening in my body, learn how to take care of myself, and come back to a balanced state."

Before You Begin

There are a few tips that are helpful to consider before you practice. The main thing is not to eat immediately beforehand. Having a full stomach can make some of the practices uncomfortable. You want to be wearing clothing that you can move in freely, but you definitely do not need expensive yoga pants!

Now, decide where you want to practice. You might want to do a mat practice, which means a few different things. It can include standing, kneeling, lying on your abdomen, and lying on your back. You might be able to do some of these things and not others, which is fine. But one key question about mat practice is whether you can get down to the floor and, more importantly, get back up. Alternatively, standing poses do not require getting up and down from the floor. You can also practice in a chair or lying in bed, or a combination of all of these. For example, if you don't want to get down on the floor, you could start practicing in a chair, then stand for some poses, and finally lie on a bed for the end of the session.

If you're using a chair for your practice, choose one that is sturdy and, if possible, doesn't have arms. It can be helpful if the seat is solid rather than cushioned. If you use a wheelchair, you may want to consider transferring to a chair, if that's accessible to you. Many wheelchairs have soft, cushioned seats and backrests, which don't offer much traction or resistance. While this soft surface is helpful for long-term sitting, it's not useful in most yoga poses because you don't have a solid surface to push against as you practice.

Similarly, when practicing in a bed, try to create a firm and even surface to work from. This means moving the blankets aside and even placing a yoga mat on top of the bed. The mat can offer slightly more resistance when doing asanas. But notice how the softness of the bed can still allow for too much give. Certain poses, such as those done on your abdomen, may not be effective in bed. Practicing a prone backbend, such as Cobra Pose in bed, is not recommended because the lower back can become overly curved. It's safest to practice relatively gentle supine poses and movements, as well as side-lying poses.

One of the biggest challenges in practicing yoga is figuring out how deep to go into a pose or how long to hold it. If you go too far, then you may cause injury. If you don't put any energy into it, then you're not going to get any benefit. In the Yoga Sutras, Patanjali offers three teachings on asana practice. First he explains that asana is a steady and comfortable pose. He continues on to tell us how to practice asana: "By lessening the natural tendency for restlessness and by meditating on the infinite, posture is mastered."[1] Finally, he explains that once you are established in asana, you will transcend the duality of nature. This basically means that through cultivating balance, we find peace.

It's helpful to bring a sense of wonder and exploration to yoga practice. In fact, the state of mind that you experience in yoga practice is the same experience of flow that you get in the midst of creating art or music or dancing. To be in the flow means that you have successfully connected with the present moment and found your way back from the pain of the past and the worries of the future.

Don't underestimate the creative force within you. Learn how to practice a few poses, breathing practices, relaxation, and meditation techniques. Then let go of what you think you "should" do and allow yourself a moment of introspection. Here are a few questions you can ask yourself as you begin your practice each day:

- How do I feel emotionally and physically?
- How does my body want to move, or not want to move, right now?
- What practice would bring the most healing to my body and mind at this moment?
- What is my intention for this practice?

It's often best to enter a practice with more questions than answers. I find that many of my questions in life are resolved when I get on my mat. In the movement, flow, breath, and pause, I often discover answers that I never expected to find. You can take this one step further. If you're struggling with some big challenge or question in your life, you can use your practice to find answers. Try asking yourself the question, or write it down, before you begin to practice. Then let it go and begin to turn inward. Do your centering, movement, and relaxation, and you may be surprised by what you discover. Sometimes the busy mind interferes with messages coming through from your intuition. If you can get your mind to be quiet just for a few moments, then wisdom can flow through.

FOR YOGA TEACHERS 15

I TRUST that all yoga teachers mean well and come to the teaching of yoga out of a love for yoga and a passion for service. So now that you've learned about how to practice Accessible Yoga, it's time to think about how you can make your yoga classes truly accessible. With that in mind, I offer the following suggestions for all yoga classes.

WELCOME EVERYONE

Part of making yoga accessible is welcoming people of all abilities and backgrounds to your classes. The first step is to consider your publicity materials—the imagery and language you use to describe your classes. It's essential to be clear in your class descriptions about what kind of practices are included: Is the class open to all levels? Can people practice in chairs? Do you use music?

Getting this information in advance allows potential students to be more prepared for what they will experience, which evokes a feeling of safety when they come to class. This is also the first step in trauma-informed teaching, providing students with clear information about what they'll be doing in your class.

It's also important to consider how to make your classes financially accessible. Can you offer sliding-scale pricing or scholarships? You might explore financial support for your classes from nonprofits involved with yoga; from associations that are dedicated to the populations you serve (such as the National Multiple Sclerosis Society); or from the organization that sponsors the classes (yoga studio, religious organization, corporate sponsor). For many people, the price of drop-in yoga classes is out of reach, yet everyone deserves access to these teachings.

INVITE ALL STUDENTS TO PARTICIPATE IN ALL PRACTICES

During class, make sure no one is simply left out because you don't know how to adapt to their needs. Each student can be included in a conscious way, even if his or her movement is limited. The key is finding a way to teach multiple levels at the same time.

To do this, try to consider each practice as a spectrum of possibilities instead of a static pose. Rather than approach an asana by teaching one form, focus on the overarching goal and benefits (and even contraindications) of that practice. From this deeper understanding, your students can learn to explore multiple variations.

For example, rather than teach a version of Shoulderstand as the "full expression of the pose," first consider the benefits of Shoulderstand, which include resting the heart, strengthening the core muscles, and improving lymphatic drainage and venous blood flow. Then consider how you can find those qualities at whatever level the student is practicing—whether it's in a chair, on a mat, or even standing.

If you have a new student and don't know what his or her ability is, try a more collaborative approach. Offer suggestions and encourage self-exploration and self-awareness. In fact, the first thing to do with new students is to teach them *how* to practice rather than jumping into specific practices. This means explaining some basic concepts that define yoga—that it's an inward, noncompetitive practice.

We also need to teach students that pain is a sign that they've gone too far. Of course, some people have chronic pain and need to be extra-sensitive to that experience. Also, some students may have paralysis and not be able to feel sensations in a part of their bodies, so there isn't any pain to help them regulate their movement. For those students, it's best to spend time exploring safe movements in a private setting before joining a group class. Also, with a new student it's always useful to talk about not competing in yoga and about really trying to step back from the edge, that place where challenge turns into pain.

Offering variations at different levels is key to making a class accessible and integrated. This means that teachers need to learn how to teach for multiple levels of physical ability at the same time. I like to think of an accessible yoga class like a jazz ensemble; each student is like a musician playing a riff on a common theme, and the teacher is the conductor. It may look chaotic and seem like everyone is doing their own thing, but there is a harmony running through the entire group. This can be a difficult skill to develop, but it is one that teachers can cultivate over time.

When teaching a multiple-level class, try to find a way to bring all students together for a portion of each practice, even if they're practicing in a way that looks completely different. One way is to set up students in each version of a pose separately; for example, set up on the mat first and then in a chair. Then give some common instruction about how to come into the pose together. This creates an opportunity for multiple levels of a pose to be done in different ways simultaneously.

For example, you can teach chair and mat versions of Cobra Pose at the same time. Bring the students on the mat into a preparatory position with their foreheads on the floor, then bring the students in chairs into a preparatory position with their heads lowered. Now bring all the students into the pose together using common instructions that work for both. Something like, "Exhale, grounding down, then inhale and lengthen your neck, slowly curling up your head, neck, and chest." If this is too complicated, at least find a moment when everyone is in their own version of the pose and they can all breath together. Continually reconnecting the group in this way creates a feeling of inclusivity, equity, and community in the class.

You can also demonstrate one version and verbally teach a different one. If you are teaching chair and mat versions of a pose simultaneously, tell the students in the chairs to watch you as you demonstrate and give verbal cues to the students on the mat. This can be challenging to do, so be patient with yourself.

Another option is to have an assistant demonstrate one variation of a pose while you teach a different variation. I would be cautious about using students as models in this way. It's not a student's job to demonstrate for the group, unless you have discussed it with the student previously, and they are interested in assisting you in this way.

Finally, when setting up the classroom, try to make sure that everyone feels like a part of the group. Students practicing in chairs or wheelchairs can be lined up with other students equally. In fact, students practicing in chairs often benefit from having a yoga mat under the chairs for additional traction. Physically including everyone in the "circle" of students sends an important message that everyone is equal, rather than creating a subtle hierarchy through placement and space.

As a teacher, your positive attention is a powerful tool. There needs to be an equal share of love for everyone in the room, not just the "advanced" students. Sometimes getting out of the house and coming to class is a huge success for someone with a disability or chronic illness. Be careful about always praising physical ability over other forms of ability and effort. What is the goal of yoga anyway—gymnastics or peace of mind? Can you praise the fact that someone with chronic fatigue made it to class today? Or can you praise someone for coming out of a pose early and acknowledging their own limit?

CONSENT

Touching students without consent is always unacceptable. In public, drop-in yoga classes, teachers usually don't know each students' individual medical history and their past experience with trauma. This makes adjustments questionable even with consent. Also, understanding the scope of practice for a yoga teacher is essential before offering touch. Are you adequately trained to offer adjustments?

According to the International Association of Yoga Therapists, adjustments aren't in the scope of practice of yoga therapists, even those with more than a thousand hours of training. Is it legal in your state according to your level of training? In some states, it is only legal to touch a client or student if you are medical personnel, a licensed massage therapist, or clergy.

There are a variety of ways to make touch optional in your classes. First, you can give a general announcement at the beginning of the session, telling students that they have the right to decline to be touched during the class and giving them the tools to do so. For example, you can use consent cards, which students can turn to one side to say they want touch or the other side to say they don't want touch. However, consent cards may not work well with chair yoga students or those who are visually impaired. And consent cards are just one step in this process.

There are three important qualities of consent: informed, ongoing, and enthusiastic.

Informed consent means the students actually understand what you're asking them to consent to. For example, asking students simply, "Can I give you an adjustment in that pose?" is not enough information for them to decide if they want to be touched. Instead, say something specific like, "Can I touch your right arm to help you lift it up?"

Ongoing consent means that just because a student gives you consent at one point in the class doesn't mean that you have consent to touch at another time. So you need to continue to get consent each time you touch students, regardless of their previous affirmative response. Ongoing consent means that we open up a dialogue with our students during class. This is in contrast to the silent obedience that is the earmark of certain yoga classes. You can create an environment where declining touch is accepted and even celebrated, where students are learning to connect with themselves and speak up for what they need.

Enthusiastic consent means that you need a clear, affirmative response when requesting to touch a student. Remember, as the teacher, you are in the power position in this relationship, and students may defer to your judgment even if they don't fully agree with what's happening. That's why these guidelines are essential for creating a safe environment in yoga class.

If you feel like you have too many students in a group class to achieve this type of consent, you may need to avoid touching your students, get assistants, or teach smaller classes. Also, it may be more challenging to get consent to touch students who speak a different language than you, who don't use words to speak, or who have dementia or Alzheimer's disease. In those cases, it's best to avoid touch or work with the person's care team to come up with effective communication tools.

COLLABORATION AND CREATIVITY

Support students in developing their own self-awareness through their personal exploration of yoga practices. This can be done by constantly emphasizing their own experience versus what you think they are experiencing. If you teach a practice and say that it's calming, what happens if some students don't find it calming? Does that mean their experience is invalid? How do they reconcile their own experience with the experience you want them to have?

Shifting the focus to personal exploration rather than goal orientation is another way to make the class more of a collaborative experience. De-emphasizing the "full expression of the pose" and not working toward a "peak pose" will allow the students to find their own practice.

Encourage your students' creativity instead. Teach them to approach every practice as a new opportunity, bringing fresh eyes and an open mind rather than relying on past experience. Instead of building a practice based on what they "should" experience, creativity means that they are open to what is happening now. Creativity is the earmark of spirituality, and it can only happen within a safe, supportive environment.

Remind your students that yoga is a spiritual practice, and everyone shares that same spiritual essence equally, regardless of what they look like or what they can do. You don't have to use the word *spiritual* to do this. You can talk about essence, consciousness, wholeness, et cetera. It's so easy to get competitive with asana practice and think that more is better. Always remember that outer ability does not equal inner peace.

An important part of yoga is learning to befriend yourself and quiet the inner conflict in your mind. That inner cease-fire comes through acceptance and self-love, not necessarily through gymnastic ability and outer achievement.

SELF-CARE AND COMMUNITY BUILDING

The goal of teaching yoga is to empower your students to find peace of mind through their own practice and not to become reliant on you. Encourage them to build a home practice, even if it starts very slowly. To do this, teach general concepts regarding how and why we practice. Empowerment also comes from being told that we're worthy of self-care.

Interestingly, community building goes along with self-care. Many people are isolated and don't have a community. This can lead to a reduction in healthy lifestyle choices and even self-destructive behavior. Yoga classes can act as social networks, and many people need that kind of support.

Can you spend time helping to build those social connections? Here are a few simple ways to do so. Have the students introduce themselves at the beginning or end of every class. Spend a few minutes checking in at the beginning of class and asking people how they are doing. Spend a few minutes after class socializing and encouraging the students to talk to each other. Maybe offer tea or a snack after class.

"Taking yoga off the mat" means to come from a place of love, which is known as service, or karma yoga. We have the opportunity to practice karma yoga when we're teaching. Teaching from a place of love can simply mean putting the students' best interests first and considering what would be most beneficial for them. It also means being kind, patient, and loving in our approach and demeanor.

Working on all these levels, we can begin to open the practice of yoga to people of all abilities. What's so powerful in this accessible approach is that by using it, we simultaneously open our own minds to a deeper understanding of the meaning of yoga. We experience the truth of yoga—that it is a pathway to connect with our true self. This true self resides in all of us, regardless of our physical ability, past trauma, bank account, race, gender identity, or any kind of identity.

It's not a question of including people who are usually left out; it's about understanding the truth behind all these labels: we are ultimately all made of that same essence. Like I always say, yoga is not about having a flexible body, it's about having a flexible mind, a mind that is clear enough for the truth to shine through.

APPENDIX

Sample Practices

MIXED SESSION (CHAIR/WALL/MAT) LONG #1

CHAIR

STANDING

MAT

CHAIR

Mixed Session (Chair/Wall/Mat) Long #2

Chair

Standing

Mat

Chair

Mixed Session (Chair/Wall/Mat) Short #1

Chair

Standing

Mat

Mixed Session (Chair/Wall/Mat) Short #2

Chair

Standing

Mat

Accessible Yoga
(www.accessibleyoga.org)

Accessible Yoga is an international grassroots, nonprofit organization dedicated to sharing yoga with everyone. It offers conferences around the world to provide networking and education opportunities to yoga teachers. It also focuses on connecting its huge network of Accessible Yoga Ambassadors around the world. It has more than twenty regional groups with more than ten languages, helping to increase awareness and provide information about making yoga accessible.

Accessible Yoga Training
(www.accessibleyogatraining.com)

Accessible Yoga offers training for yoga teachers, health care professionals, and experienced students in making yoga accessible to everyone. The program focuses on how to adapt basic yoga practices for students practicing on a mat, in a chair, standing, or in bed. It also emphasizes a creative and collaborative approach to make all students feel comfortable in group yoga classes and provides teachers with tools for leading multiple-level classes, where no one is left out.

ORGANIZATIONS

Abundant Well Being
(www.abundantwellbeing.com)

This organization offers international workshops and teacher training, with a focus on expressing yoga and its subtle uses for spiritual growth and complete healing.

Access 2 Yoga (www.access2yoga.com)

This Chicago-based organization holds adaptive yoga classes, workshops, and trainings for students and yoga teachers who would like to provide accessible yoga instruction to students of all abilities.

Amplify and Activate Summit
(www.amplifyandactivate.com)

This summit is focused on racial justice and building trust, bringing together teachers who are actively using their practice of yoga to lead social justice movements.

Asanas for Autism and Special Needs
(www.asanasforautismandspecialneeds.com)

This organization gives classes and teacher training to bring yoga to children of all abilities.

Ashrams for Autism
(www.ashrams4autism.org)

Founded in 2010, this organization provides yoga to people of all ages and everywhere on the autism spectrum, as well as teacher training.

Black Yoga Teachers Alliance
(www.blackyogateachersalliance.org)

This organization supports black yoga teachers and practitioners.

Body Positive Yoga
(www.bodypositiveyoga.com)

In addition to offering online resources and teacher training, the Body Positive Clubhouse includes online classes for all bodies and abilities.

Buddha Body Yoga
(www.buddhabodyyoganyc.com)

Teachers adapt yoga "for larger, overweight or injured people to successfully practice." Located in New York City, the organization's live-stream classes are available every Saturday morning.

Connected Warriors
(www.connectedwarriors.org)

This organization provides evidence-based trauma-conscious yoga therapy programs for service members, veterans, and their families.

Deaf Yoga Foundation
(www.deafyoga.org)

This nonprofit provides classes, training, and advocacy to increase access to yoga to the Deaf and Hard of Hearing community.

Get Fit Where You Sit
(www.getfitwhereyousit.com)

This site provides chair yoga classes and teacher training.

Give Back Yoga Foundation
(www.givebackyoga.org)

The foundation's mission is to "support and fund certified teachers in all traditions to offer the teachings of yoga to underserved and under-resourced socio-economic segments of the community."

Integral Yoga
(www.integralyoga.org)

This international organization is dedicated to the classical teachings of yoga.

International Association of Yoga Therapists
(www.iayt.org)

This association creates standards and conferences for yoga therapists.

Kidding Around Yoga
(www.kiddingaroundyoga.com)

This program provides KAY yoga teacher training, including Accessible Yoga for children.

Liberation Prison Yoga
(www.liberationprisonyoga.com)

This organization brings yoga to incarcerated individuals.

Love Your Brain Foundation
(www.loveyourbrain.com)

The foundation supports people who have experienced traumatic brain injuries and their caregivers to participate in free yoga programs.

Mind Body Solutions
(www.mindbodysolutions.org)

This nonprofit organization offers training and workshops on adapting yoga for persons living with disabilities.

New Leaf Foundation
(www.newleafyoga.org)

This organization supports youth from marginalized communities in Ontario, Canada.

Off the Mat, Into the World
(www.offthematintotheworld.org)

A nonprofit organization dedicated to training leaders around the world in social change, Off the Mat, Into the World works to be the bridge between yoga, self-inquiry, and effective community action.

OG Yoga
(www.ogyoga.org)

OG Yoga offers trauma-informed yoga in the San Diego area.

Piedmont Yoga Community
(www.piedmontyogacommunity.org)

This organization provides classes and teacher training in yoga for people with disabilities in Oakland, California.

Prison Yoga Project
(www.prisonyoga.org)

Teachers promote the peace, health, and well-being of people in the criminal justice system and those supporting them.

SunLight Chair Yoga
(www.sunlightchairyoga.com)

Chair yoga classes and online teacher training are offered through this site.

Therapeutic Yoga
(www.therapeuticyoga.com)

This company makes teacher training, classes, and workshops on the healing aspects of yoga available.

Three and a Half Acres
(www.threeandahalfacres.org)

This nonprofit provides yoga, breathing, and mindfulness techniques to underserved communities in New York City, using these tools to support individuals in recognizing their own power for positive change.

Trauma Center Trauma Sensitive Yoga
(www.traumasensitiveyoga.org)

Yoga teachers and mental health professionals can train to provide empirically validated, clinical intervention for complex trauma or chronic, treatment-resistant, post-traumatic stress disorder (PTSD).

Uprising Yoga
(www.uprisingyoga.org)

Founded in 2011, URY brings yoga to incarcerated youth and provides trauma-informed teacher training.

Warriors at Ease
(www.warriorsatease.org)

This organization uses yoga to support the health and healing of service members, veterans, and their families.

Yoga Alliance
(www.yogaalliance.org)

This is an international registry for yoga teachers and teacher training programs, with a directory of schools and teachers.

Yoga & Body Image Coalition
(www.ybicoalition.com)

This coalition promotes yoga that is accessible, body positive, and reflects the full range of human diversity. It includes a critical social justice component by challenging industry leaders and media creators to expand their vision of what a yogi looks like.

Yoga for Amputees
(www.yogaforamputees.com)

This company offers resources, classes, and teacher training on yoga for amputees.

Yoga for Arthritis
(www.arthritis.yoga)

This site offers information about the benefits of yoga for people living with arthritis, as well as teacher training and a teacher directory.

Yoga for the Special Child
(www.specialyoga.com)

This multilevel, comprehensive program of yoga techniques is designed to enhance the natural development of children with special needs.

Yoga International
(www.yogainternational.com)

Yoga International is an online resource for articles and classes.

YogaMate

(www.yogamate.org)

This site has online resources for yoga teachers and therapists.

Yoga Moves MS

(www.yogamovesms.org)

This nonprofit is dedicated to providing therapeutic yoga to individuals with MS and neuromuscular conditions in small group classes throughout southeastern Michigan.

Yoga of 12-Step Recovery

(www.y12sr.com)

The teacher training and resources here integrate yoga somatics and twelve-step recovery.

Yoga of Recovery

(www.yogaofrecovery.com)

This organization's training and retreats integrate the wisdom of yoga and Ayurveda with the tools of twelve-step recovery.

YogaReach

(www.yoga-reach.org)

YogaReach instructors teach a specialized system of poses, balance and strengthening activities, and mindful breathing techniques for people with Parkinson's disease and other neurological diseases.

Yoga Service Council

(www.yogaservicecouncil.org)

The aim of this organization is to maximize the effectiveness, sustainability, and impact of those working to make yoga and mindfulness equally accessible to all by offering conferences, membership, and a best practices series.

Yoga Therapy in Cancer and Chronic Illness

(www.ycatyogaincancer.com)

The YCat program trains teachers to adapt yoga for people with cancer and other chronic or life-threatening illnesses.

Yogasteya

(www.yogasteya.com)

This online yoga class platform is for people of all shapes, sizes, and abilities.

Books

Austin, Miriam. *Yoga for Wimps, Poses for the Flexibility Impaired.* New York City: Sterling Publishing, 2000.

Berila, Beth, Melanie Klein, and Chelsea Jackson Roberts. *Yoga, the Body, and Embodied Social Change: An Intersectional Feminist Analysis.* Lanham, MD: Lexington Books, 2016.

Bell, Baxter, and Nina Zolotow. *Yoga for Healthy Aging: A Guide to Lifelong Well-Being.* Boulder, CO: Shambhala Publications, 2017.

Bondy, Dianne. *Yoga for Everyone: 50 Poses for Every Type of Body.* Indianapolis, IN: DK Publishing, 2019.

Bryant, Edwin F. *The Yoga Sutras of Patanjali: A New Edition, Translation, and Commentary.* New York City: North Point Press, 2009.

Byrom, Thomas. *The Heart of Awareness: A Translation of the Ashtavakra Gita.* Boston, MA: Shambhala Publications, 2001.

Byron, Erin, and Steffany Moonaz. *Yoga Therapy for Arthritis.* London, UK: Singing Dragon, 2018.

Carrera, Jaganath. *Awakening: Inside Yoga Meditation.* Woodland Park, NJ: Yoga Life Publications, 2012.

———. *Inside the Yoga Sutras.* Yogaville, VA: Integral Yoga Publications, 2006.

Christensen, Alice. *The American Yoga Association's Easy Does It Yoga: The Safe and Gentle Way to Health and Well-Being.* New York City: Fireside, 1999.

Clampett, Cheri, and Biff Mithoefer. *The Therapeutic Yoga Kit: Sixteen Postures for Self-Healing through*

Quiet Yin Awareness. Rochester, VT: Healing Arts Press, 2009.

Danzig, Marsha. *Yoga for Amputees.* Dayton, OH: Sacred Oak Publishing, 2018.

Devi, Nischala Joy. *The Healing Path of Yoga: Time-Honored Wisdom and Scientifically Proven Methods That Alleviate Stress, Open Your Heart, and Enrich Your Life.* New York City: Three Rivers Press, 2000.

———. *The Secret Power of Yoga: A Woman's Guide to the Heart and Spirit of the Yoga Sutras.* New York City: Three Rivers Press, 2007.

Dooreck, Stacie. *Sunlight Chair Yoga: Yoga for Everyone!* Ross, CA: Sunlight Yoga Publishers, 2014.

Eisenberg, Mindy. *Adaptive Yoga Moves Any Body.* N.p.: Orange Cat Press, 2015.

Farhi, Donna. *The Breathing Book: Good Health and Vitality Through Essential Breathwork.* New York City: Owl Books, 1998.

———. *Teaching Yoga: Exploring the Teacher-Student Relationship.* Berkeley, CA: Rodmell Press, 2006.

Feuerstein, Georg. *The Yoga Tradition: Its History, Literature, Philosophy and Practice.* Prescott, AZ: Hohm Press, 2001.

Fishman, Loren M., and Eric L. Small. *Yoga and Multiple Sclerosis: A Journey to Health and Healing.* New York City: Demos Medical Publishing, 2007.

Frankl, Viktor. *Man's Search for Meaning.* New York City: Simon & Schuster, 1984.

Gates, Rolf. *Meditations from the Mat: Daily Reflections on the Path of Yoga.* New York City: Anchor Books, 2002.

Guest-Jelley, Anna. *Curvy Yoga: Love Yourself and Your Body a Little More Each Day.* New York City: Sterling Publishing Co., 2017.

Hendrickson, Peter. *Alive and Well: A Path for Living in a Time of HIV.* New York City: Irvington Publishers, 1990.

Horton, Carol, ed. *Best Practices for Yoga in the Criminal Justice System.* Atlanta, GA: YSC–Omega Publications, 2017.

———. *Best Practices for Yoga with Veterans.* Atlanta, GA: YSC–Omega Publications, 2016.

Isherwood, Christopher, and Swami Prabhavananda. *How to Know God: The Yoga Aphorisms of Patanjali.* Hollywood, CA: Vedanta Society of Southern California, 1981.

Johnson, Michelle Cassandra. *Skill in Action: Radicalizing Your Yoga Practice to Create a Just World.* Portland, OR: Radical Transformation Media, 2017.

Kaminoff, Leslie, and Amy Matthews. *Yoga Anatomy.* Champaign, IL: Human Kinetics, 2012.

Keil, David. *Functional Anatomy of Yoga: A Guide for Practitioners and Teachers.* Chichester, UK: Lotus Publishing, 2014.

Kerr, Meera Patricia. *Big Yoga: A Simple Guide for Bigger Bodies.* Garden City Park, NY: Square One Publishers, 2010.

Klein, Melanie. *Yoga Rising: 30 Empowering Stories from Yoga Renegades for Every Body.* Woodbury, MN: Llewelyn Publications, 2018.

Klein, Melanie, and Anna Guest-Jelley. *Yoga and Body Image: 25 Personal Stories about Beauty, Bravery & Loving Your Body.* Woodbury, MN: Llewelyn Publications, 2014.

Lasater, Judith Hanson. *Restore and Rebalance: Yoga for Deep Relaxation.* Boulder, CO: Shambhala Publications, 2017.

Levine, Stephen. *Healing into Life and Death.* New York City: Anchor Books, 1987.

Lipton, Lauren. *Yoga Bodies: Real People, Real Stories & the Power of Transformation.* San Francisco: Chronicle Books, 2017.

Mandelkorn, Philip. *To Know Your Self: The Essential Teachings of Swami Satchidananda.* Yogaville, VA: Integral Yoga Publications, 2008.

Miller, Richard. *Yoga Nidra: A Meditative Practice for Deep Relaxation and Healing.* Boulder, CO: Sounds True Inc, 2010.

Nair, Camella. *Aqua Kriya Yoga: Making Yoga Accessible.* Bloomington, IL: Authorhouse, 2007.

Ornish, Dean. *Love and Survival: The Scientific Basis for the Healing Power of Intimacy.* New York City: Harper Collins, 1998.

Porges, Stephen W. *The Pocket Guide to the Polyvagal*

Theory: The Transformative Power of Feeling Safe. New York City: W. W. Norton & Co., 2017.

Remski, Matthew. *Practice and All Is Coming: Abuse, Cult Dynamics, and Healing in Yoga and Beyond.* Rangiora, New Zealand: Embodied Wisdom Publications, 2019.

Rosen, Richard. *The Yoga of Breath: A Step-by-Step Guide to Pranayama.* Boston, MA: Shambhala Publications, 2002.

Rossman, Martin. *Healing Yourself: A Step-By-Step Program for Better Health through Imagery.* New York City: Walker Publishing, 1987.

Sanford, Matthew. *Waking: A Memoir of Trauma and Transcendence.* Emmaus, PA: Rodale Books, 2006.

Satchidananda, Swami. *The Living Gita: The Complete Bhagavad Gita.* Buckingham, VA: Integral Yoga Publications, 1988.

———. *The Yoga Sutras of Patanjali: Translation and Commentary by Sri Swami Satchidananda.* Buckingham, VA: Integral Yoga Publications, 1978.

Schatz, Mary Pullig. *Back Care Basics: A Doctor's Gentle Yoga Program for Back and Neck Pain Relief.* Berkeley, CA: Rodmell Press, 1992.

Singleton, Mark. *Yoga Body: The Origins of Modern Posture Practice.* New York City: Oxford University Press, 2010.

Sivananda, Swami. *Bliss Divine: A Book of Spiritual Essays on the Lofty Purpose of Human Life and the Means to Its Achievement.* Uttarakhand, India, 2013

———. *Thought Power.* Uttaranchal, India: Divine Life Society, 2004.

Sparrowe, Linda, and Patricia Walden. *The Woman's Book of Yoga and Health: A Lifelong Guide to Wellness.* Boston, MA: Shambhala Publications, 2002.

Stanley, Jessamyn. *Every Body Yoga: Let Go of Fear, Get on the Mat, Love Your Body.* New York City: Workman Publishing, 2017.

Stone, Michael. *The Inner Tradition of Yoga: A Guide to Yoga Philosophy for the Contemporary Practitioner.* Boston, MA: Shambhala Publications, 2008.

Swanson, Ann. *Science of Yoga.* London, UK: Dorling Kindersley Publishing, 2019.

Vivekananda, Swami. *Raja Yoga.* New York City: Ramakrishna Vivekananda Center, 1982.

Weintraub, Amy. *Yoga for Depression: A Compassionate Guide to Relieve Suffering through Yoga.* New York City: Broadway Books, 2004.

White, David Gordon. *The Yoga Sutra of Patanjali: A Biography.* Princeton, NJ: Princeton University Press, 2014.

Wittstamm, Willem. *The Best Is Yet to Come: Aging Gracefully with Yoga50plus.* Clenze, Germany: www.yoga50plus.de, 2016.

Introduction: My Story

1. D. Ornish et al., "Can Lifestyle Changes Reverse Coronary Heart Disease?" *The Lancet* 336, no. 8708 (1990): 129–33, www.thelancet.com/journals/lancet/article/PII0140-6736(90)91656-U/abstract.

2. Coleman Barks, trans., *The Essential Rumi* (England: Castle Books, 1997), 155–56.

3. Seth Powell, "The Ancient Yoga Strap: A Brief History of the Yogapatta," *The Luminescent*, June 16, 2018, www.theluminescent.org/2018/06/the-ancient-yoga-strap-yogapatta.html.

4. Matthew Remski, "WAWADIA: A Working Thesis," Matthew Remski blog, November 4, 2014, http://matthewremski.com/wordpress/wawadia-a-working-thesis.

Chapter 1: Accessible Yoga Philosophy

1. United Nations—Disability, "Convention on the Rights of Persons with Disabilities (CRPD)," accessed January 29, 2018, www.un.org/development/desa/disabilities/convention-on-the-rights-of-persons-with-disabilities.html.

2. Swami Satchidananda, *The Living Gita: The Complete Bhagavad Gita* (Buckingham, VA: Integral Yoga Publications, 1988), 91–92.

3. Michelle Cassandra Johnson, *Skill in Action: Radicalizing Your Yoga Practice to Create a Just World* (Portland, OR: Radical Transformation Media, 2018), 31.

4. Jochen Gebauer et al., "Mind-Body Practices and the Self: Yoga and Meditation Do Not Quiet the Ego, but Instead Boost Self-Enhancement," *Psychological Science* 29, no. 8 (2018): 1299–1308, https://eprints.soton.ac.uk/420273.

5. Seth Powell, trans., *The Yogasūtras of Patañjali* (digital text for online course "YS 201: Classical Yoga," Yogic Studies, 2018).

6. From *The Heart of Awareness: A Translation of the Ashtavakra Gita*, by Thomas Byrom, 1–3, ©2001. Reprinted by arrangement with Shambhala Publications, Inc., Boulder, CO. www.shambhala.com.

7. Swami Satchidananda, *The Yoga Sutras of Patanjali* (Buckingham, VA: Integral Yoga Publications, 1990), 146.

Chapter 2: A Revolutionary Practice

1. Seth Powell, trans., *The Yogasūtras of Patañjali* (digital text for online course "YS 201: Classical Yoga," Yogic Studies, 2018).

2. Jill Miller, "Inside My Injury: How I Ended Up with a Total Hip Replacement at Age 45," *Yoga Journal*, July 11, 2018, www.yogajournal.com/lifestyle/inside-my-injury-how-i-ended-up-with-a-total-hip-replacement-at-age-45.

3. Theo Wildcroft, "Post-lineage Yoga," April 20, 2016, www.wildyoga.co.uk/2018/04/post-lineage-yoga.

4. Swami Satchidananda, *The Yoga Sutras of Patanjali* (Buckingham, VA: Integral Yoga Publications, 1990), 19.

5. Marlysa B. Sullivan et al., "Yoga Therapy and Polyvagal Theory: The Convergence of Traditional Wisdom and Contemporary Neuroscience for Self-Regulation

and Resistance," *Frontiers in Human Neuroscience* 12 (2018): 67, www.frontiersin.org/articles/10.3389/fnhum.2018.00067/full.

6. D. Ornish et al., "Can Lifestyle Changes Reverse Coronary Heart Disease?" *The Lancet* 336, no. 8708 (1990): 129–33, www.thelancet.com/journals/lancet/article/PII0140-6736(90)91656-U/abstract.

7. Sue McGreevey, "Eight Weeks to a Better Brain," *The Harvard Gazette*, January 21, 2011, https://news.harvard.edu/gazette/story/2011/01/eight-weeks-to-a-better-brain.

8. Jim Sliwa, "Yoga Effective at Reducing Symptoms of Depression," American Psychological Association, August 3, 2017, www.apa.org/news/press/releases/2017/08/yoga-depression.aspx.

9. Frontiers, "Yoga and Meditation Improve Mind-Body Health and Stress Resilience," *Science Daily*, August 22, 2017, www.sciencedaily.com/releases/2017/08/170822104855.htm.

10. Jesmy Jose and Maria Martin Joseph, "Imagery: It's Effects and Benefits on Sports Performance and Psychological Variables: A Review Study," *International Journal of Physiology, Nutrition and Physical Education* 3, no. 2 (2018): 190–93, www.journalofsports.com/pdf/2018/vol3issue2/PartE/3-2-41-617.pdf.

Chapter 3: Warming Up

1. The Krishna Path, "Did Quantum Physics Come from the Vedas?" Uplift, July 21, 2016, https://upliftconnect.com/quantum-physics-vedas.

Chapter 7: Backward Bending

1. E. G. Culham, H. A. Jimenez, and C. E. King, "Thoracic Kyphosis, Rib Mobility, and Lung Volumes in Normal Women and Women with Osteoporosis," *Spine* 19, no. 11 (1994): 1250–51, www.ncbi.nlm.nih.gov/pubmed/8073317.

2. Pauline Anderson, "Yoga as Good as Physical Therapy for Back Pain," Medscape, September 29, 2016, www.medscape.com/viewarticle/869487#vp_2.

Chapter 12: Breathing

1. Swami Satchidananda, *The Yoga Sutras of Patanjali* (Buckingham, VA: Integral Yoga Publications, 1990), 163.

2. A. Price and R. Eccles, "Nasal Airflow and Brain Activity: Is There a Link?" *Journal of Laryngology and Otology* 130, no. 9 (2016): 794–99, www.ncbi.nlm.nih.gov/pubmed/27477330.

Chapter 13: Meditating

1. Swami Satchidananda, *The Yoga Sutras of Patanjali* (Buckingham, VA: Integral Yoga Publications, 1990), 19.

2. Satchidananda, *The Yoga Sutras of Patanjali*, 124–25.

3. Satchidananda, *The Yoga Sutras of Patanjali*, 171.

Chapter 14: Building a Home Practice

1. Swami Satchidananda, *The Yoga Sutras of Patanjali* (Buckingham, VA: Integral Yoga Publications, 1990), 154.

PHOTOGRAPHER

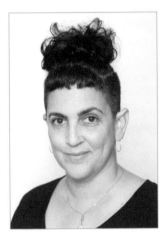

Sarit Z. Rogers

Sarit Z. Rogers is a photographer and founder of the LoveMore Movement. She's also a Somatic Experiencing® Practitioner, a community partner in the Yoga and Body Image Coalition, an Accessible Yoga Ambassador, a writer, and a practitioner of the dharma. She found emotional freedom and the ability to love herself through the practices of yoga, meditation, and SE™. She found the courage to speak the truth through writing and photography. It was on the mat where she learned how to climb safely back into her body; it was on paper where she found her wings and learned how to fly. She shares these practices with adolescents in treatment, adults recovering from trauma, and incarcerated people. Her work can be found on the covers of the books *21st Century Yoga*, *Yoga Ph.D.*, *Yoga and Body Image*, and *Yoga Rising: 30 Inspiring Stories from Yoga Renegades for Every Body*; in *LA Yoga* magazine; and featured on the Yoga International website, among others. www.saritphotography.com, www.saritzrogers.com

CONTRIBUTORS

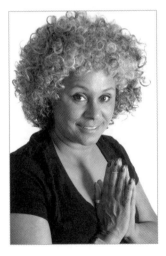

De Jur Jones

De Jur has been a yoga devotee since 2001. She attended Loyola Marymount University's yoga therapy program and currently teaches victim-centered, trauma-informed yoga to commercially sexually exploited children with UpRising Yoga. Serving this population sparked an interest to learn everything she could about trauma, how it affects victims and survivors, and how yoga can help with embodiment, self-regulation, and healing. She found her niche serving under-resourced and highly traumatized communities that show up with a myriad of emotional, physical, and psychological damage. De Jur also teaches therapeutic, accessible yoga to seniors and foster care youth. Through Prison Yoga Project and Prison Yoga+Meditation, she teaches incarcerated adults. De Jur is a contributor to the Yoga Service Council's best practices book series *Best Practices for Yoga in the Criminal Justice System*. www.idreaminyoga.com

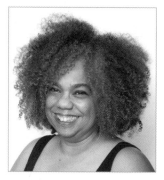

Natalie Dunbar

Natalie Dunbar is a yoga teacher who focuses on sharing the benefits of Hatha Yoga as a peaceful yet powerful way to reconnect mind, body, and spirit. Whether teaching one-on-one private sessions or by request for group classes or sports teams, Natalie teaches body positive, all-inclusive yoga for all shapes, sizes, and abilities. In addition to helping bring balance to those dealing with the stressors of everyday life, Natalie is also passionate about sharing the benefits of engaging in a regular asana practice with trauma survivors, using yoga as a vehicle on the road to healing. www.nataliedunbar.com

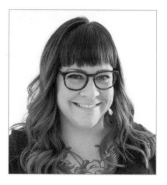

Amber Karnes

Amber Karnes is the founder of Body Positive Yoga. She's a ruckus maker, yoga teacher, social justice advocate, and a lifelong student of her body. She is the creator of the Body Positive Clubhouse, the co-creator of Yoga For All teacher training, an Accessible Yoga Trainer, and a contributor to Yoga International and the Yoga and Body Image Coalition. Through workshops, retreats, teacher training, and online offerings, she seeks to further the message of inclusivity, consent, agency, body sovereignty, and accessibility for all (on and off the yoga mat). www.bodypositiveyoga.com

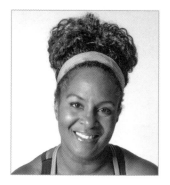

Dianne Bondy

Dianne is the author of the book *Yoga for Everyone* and a frequent contributor to Yoga International, DoYouYoga, Yoga Girl, and Omstars. She has been featured in publications such as *The Guardian*, *Huffington Post*, *Cosmopolitan*, and *People*. Dianne's commitment to increasing diversity in yoga has been recognized in her work with Pennington's, Gaiam, and the Yoga and Body Image Coalition, as well as in speaking engagements at Princeton and the University of California–Berkeley on yoga, race, and diversity. Her writing has been published in *Yoga and Body Image*, *Yoga Rising: 30 Inspiring Stories from Yoga Renegades for Every Body*, and *Yes! Yoga Has Curves*. www.diannebondyyoga.com

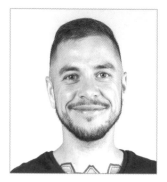

Tobias Wiggins

Tobias B. D. Wiggins, PhD, is a social justice consultant, and registered yoga teacher located in Toronto, Ontario. His lived experience as a queer and transgender man with a complex history of trauma has inspired his personal and professional yoga journey for more than twenty years. Tobias is a dedicated advocate for marginalized people, creatively combining scholarship with activism and somatic healing techniques. He teaches yoga in a way that is trauma informed, accessible to all, and fundamentally political. He aims to transform people's lives—especially those who face social injustice—by sparking internal truth and resilience. www.tobywiggins.com

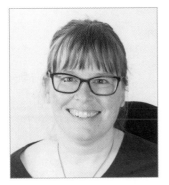

Jennifer Gasner

Jennifer has been practicing yoga since 1999 and completed her teacher training in 2014. She is passionate about integrating yoga into the lives of people with disabilities and is a member of the Accessible Yoga Advocacy Team.

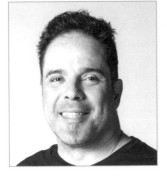

Chris Stigas

Chris suffered a spinal cord injury in 2015. After an initial recovery period, he tried physiotherapy, weight training, and suspended weight walking as methods of rehab, but when an old friend introduced him to accessible yoga practices, he started to experience recovery differently. Yoga benefits Chris by giving him the chance to participate as much as his body will allow, incorporating visualization practices when physical practices aren't available. He hopes to be able to strengthen the path from his brain through his nervous system to create more movement in his muscles. He is also the founder of HandiHelp, accessible innovations. www.handihelp.ca

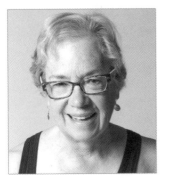

Judy Hubbell

Judy (Mirabai) Hubbell is certified as a teacher for meditation; Hatha I/II, Raja, Therapeutic, and Accessible Yoga; and T'ai Chi Chih (moving meditation). She teaches at San Francisco Integral Yoga Institute and is an instructor and previous chair of the Older Adults Department for City College of San Francisco (CCSF). Her basic class, "Body-Mind for Healthy Older Adults," uses four modalities: breath, voice, Accessible Yoga, and T'ai Chi Chih. Judy (Mirabai) loves to teach, was previously a professional singer, and taught voice for thirty-six years at Bay Area colleges (CCSF, Sonoma State University, and College of Notre Dame). She holds a master of science in music/voice from Juilliard.

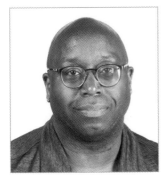

Michael Hayes

Michael created Buddha Body Yoga in 1990 as a result of his personal search for a yoga practice that suited his large physique. He is certified in Sivananda Yoga and yoga therapy, as well as through Alison West's studio, Yoga Union. He has studied extensively since 2000—primarily Iyengar, Ashtanga, Thai, and Om Vinyasa Yoga, and anatomy. Michael has more than twenty years of experience as a licensed massage therapist, spent fifteen years studying and teaching martial arts, and has performed African and modern dance. He has combined his love of dance with healing arts as a staff massage therapist for dance festivals and Broadway casts. www.buddhabodyyoganyc.com

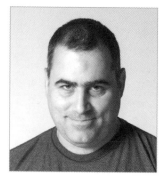

Rudra Swartz

Reverend Rudra Swartz is an ordained interfaith minister certified in Integral Yoga as a Hatha Yoga, meditation, and Raja Yoga teacher. He runs meditation workshops and intensives at the Integral Yoga Institute in New York, as well as classes in the Yoga Sutras of Patanjali, a unique class called "Judaism and Yoga: Comparative Paths," and classes in interfaith studies. He has performed wedding ceremonies in several states and has also led Jewish services in many different synagogues in many cities. He leads training for Kidding Around Yoga, a program for teaching yoga for children.

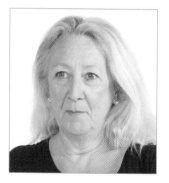

Camella Nair

Camella (Swami Nibhrtananda) has been practicing and studying yoga for decades and experienced how the practice of yoga changes over time or through illness or injury. She is certified in aquatic therapy and rehabilitation as well as being a yoga therapist, an Ayurvedic health educator, and a home funeral guide. She has authored two books on yoga and developed an accessible aqua yoga training program that caters to diverse populations. She is on the faculty at the Aquatic Therapy & Rehab Institute and bridges the gap between yoga and aquatic exercise. As a female swami, she shares deep mystical Kriya Yoga concepts with humor, enthusiasm, and a female perspective. www.camellanair.com

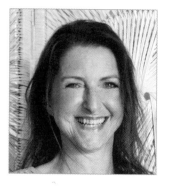

Marsha Danzig

Marsha Therese Danzig, yoga teacher, C-IAYT, RYT® 500, EdM (Harvard), is a below-knee amputee, founder of Yoga for Amputees® by Marsha T Danzig, and the author of *Yoga for Amputees: The Essential Guide to Finding Wholeness After Limb Loss*. She is a childhood bone cancer survivor, kidney transplant recipient, and one of the first amputees in the United States to teach yoga. She has more than three decades' experience as a yoga practitioner and teacher, living more than four decades as a below-knee amputee. She is the author of *From the Roots*, a breathtaking memoir about life as a survivor, spiritual seeker, and soul healer. www.yogaforamputees.com

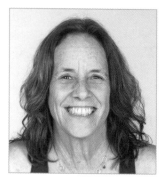

Linda Sparrowe

Linda Sparrowe is the former editor-in-chief of *Yoga International* magazine and managing editor of *Yoga Journal*. She's been instrumental in bringing the deeper practices of yoga to bear on every aspect of our lives through her talks, workshops, and retreats. Linda has lent her writing, editing, and coaching skills to a variety of projects and has authored several books, including *Yoga at Home*; *YogaMama*; *A Woman's Book of Yoga and Health*; and *Yoga: A Yoga Journal Book*. Linda is on the advisory board of the Yoga and Body Image Coalition; her talks and practices appear on yogaanytime.com and YogaUOnline, among others. She is featured in the films *Yoga Woman* and *What Is Real?* www.lindasparrowe.com

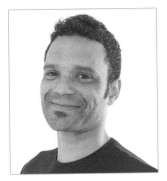

Miarco McMillian

Miarco Tiama McMillian (Hanuman) is a U.S. Marine Corps veteran. He served in Fallujah, Iraq, in 2004–2008 OIF (Operation Iraqi Freedom). Miarco renders selfless service in Los Angeles County with a focus on healing post-traumatic stress disorder and other trauma-related mental health conditions; he has taught yoga for healing PTSD in veterans' treatment facilities across California. Miarco finds healing in photography, landscaping and permaculture, yoga, and music. He is currently enrolled as a yoga therapy student in Amy Wheeler's Optimal State of Living™ program. www.selfcare-healthcare.org

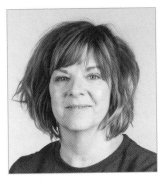

Mary-Jo Fetterly

As a senior yoga teacher, Mary-Jo teaches tantra, therapeutic, and adaptive yoga, and she advocates for a holistic approach to healing, particularly from spinal cord injury. She speaks at events about her experiences as a quadriplegic yogi and entrepreneur. Through facilitating various events on access and inclusion and serving on the Vancouver City Council Persons with Disability Advisory Committee, she is honored to be an "agent of change," helping to make our world a better place for everyone. www.mary-jo.com

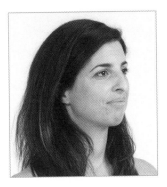

Jessica Frank

Jessica Frank is an RYT-500 Deaf yoga teacher certified in the Sivananda lineage. She is based in southern California and has been teaching yoga in American Sign Language since 2011. She has long been an advocate for access to yoga for Deaf people and is a cofacilitator of the nonprofit DeafYoga Foundation, an organization focused on sharing yoga in sign language. She holds a master's degree in cultural studies and currently teaches Deaf studies at California State University–Northridge. When she's not teaching a class, you can probably find her hiking somewhere with her Ewok-look-alike pup. www.deafyoga.org

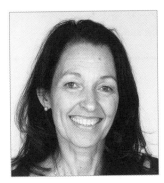

Cherie Hotchkiss

Cherie Hotchkiss, E-RYT, YACEP, created and founded Your Own Gentle Approach™. Being a certified yoga instructor prior to a diagnosis of multiple sclerosis gave her tools that have helped her manage the course of this debilitating disease. Cherie teaches her Adaptive Y.O.G.A. Workshops for the National Multiple Sclerosis Society support groups, ALS Association, the Cleveland Clinic's Lou Ruvo Center for Brain Health, Stanford School of Medicine, and local community organizations, where she helps people with challenges experience the benefits of yoga. She also teaches an experiential Y.O.G.A. Workshop for yoga instructors that allows them to experience practicing yoga with a different-ability so they can better relate to their students. Recently Cherie authored "Yoga and MS" for the National Multiple Sclerosis Society website. She is currently writing a companion guide for her workshops and producing a DVD. www.yourowngentleapproach.com

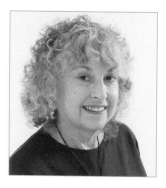

Elizabeth Wojtowicz

Elizabeth Wojtowicz is a yoga and meditation teacher; student; speaker; writer and published contributor to *Yoga Rising: 30 Inspiring Stories from Yoga Renegades for Every Body*; integrative nutrition health coach; passionate participant in the grassroots nonprofit Off the Mat, Into the World; and ability activist. She enjoys writing, going on walks, reading, art journaling, and spending time with friends and family. Her motivating mission is to continue to bring necessary awareness of yoga and meditation to people with various challenges—be they physical, emotional, or otherwise. She believes that through the practice of yoga, we have agency over our awareness. www.elayoga.weebly.com

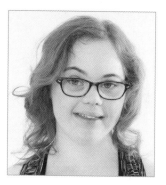

Carole Kalyani Baral

Kalyani has been a yoga teacher since graduating from the Integral Yoga Institute in New York City in 1976. A devotee of Swami Satchidananda, she taught yoga and relaxation techniques in the adult education programs in upstate New York for thirty-five years. As a board member of the North American Vegan Society, she instructed children and adult yoga and vegetarian cooking classes at the society's Summerfest conventions from 1978 to 2012. She now teaches a free accessible yoga class at the Santa Barbara Jewish Community Center for all ages and abilities. As a liver transplant recipient, she is eternally grateful for the "gift of life" she received in 2006 from a generous anonymous donor. "Service with compassion" is her motto!

Jessica Parsons

Jessica Parsons is an inclusive yoga teacher in Goleta, California. She's been teaching since she was twelve years old, and at sixteen, she began offering classes for others with special needs through the Down Syndrome Association of Santa Barbara County. She currently teaches classes for all abilities through the Santa Barbara Parks and Recreation Adapted Recreation Program. Jessica's family is made up of yoga teachers, and she has had the opportunity to attend numerous teacher trainings in basic Hatha, flow, restorative, and children's yoga through Let It Go Yoga, which her parents own. www.jessicaparsonsyoga.com

ABOUT THE AUTHOR

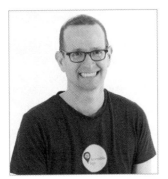 **JIVANA HEYMAN,** C-IAYT, E-RYT 500, is the founder and director of Accessible Yoga, an international nonprofit organization dedicated to increasing access to yoga teachings. He is co-owner of the Santa Barbara Yoga Center and an Integral Yoga Minister. He lives with his husband and two children in Santa Barbara, California.

Jivana has specialized in teaching yoga to people with disabilities with an emphasis on community building and social engagement. Out of this work, the Accessible Yoga organization was created to support education, training, and advocacy with the mission of shifting the public perception of yoga. In addition to offering conferences and trainings, Accessible Yoga offers a popular ambassador program with over 1,000 Accessible Yoga Ambassadors around the world.

Jivana coined the phrase "Accessible Yoga" over ten years ago, and it has now become the standard appellation for a large cross section of the immense yoga world. He brought the Accessible Yoga community together for the first time in 2015 for the Accessible Yoga Conference, which has gone on to become a focal point for this movement. There are now two conferences and over thirty-five Accessible Yoga trainings per year, as well as a strong underground yoga community supporting them.

Over the past twenty-five years, Jivana has led countless yoga teacher training programs around the world, and he dedicates his time to supporting yoga teachers who are working to serve communities that are under-represented in traditional yoga spaces. For more information, head to www .jivanaheyman.com.